ENCOUNTERING SILENCING

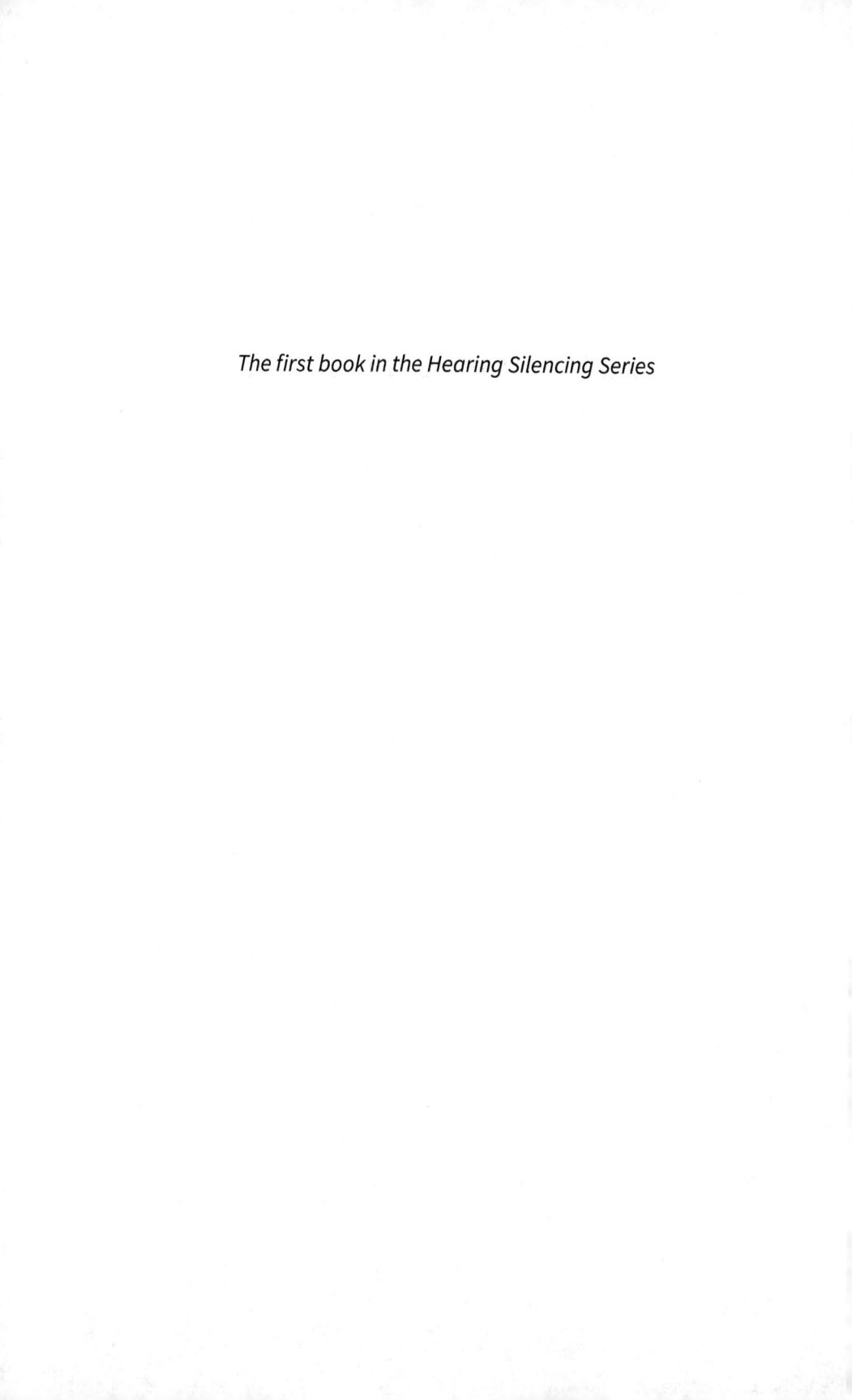

The first book in the Hearing Silencing Series

ENCOUNTERING SILENCING
Forms of Oppression
in Individuals, Families
and Communities

Edited by

Michael B. Buchholz
and Aleksandar Dimitrijević

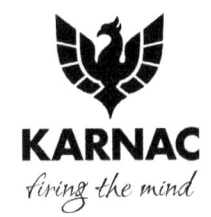

KARNAC
firing the mind

First published in 2024 by
Karnac Books Limited
62 Bucknell Road
Bicester
Oxfordshire OX26 2DS

British Library Cataloguing in Publication Data

A C.I.P. for this book is available from the British Library

ISBN: 978-1-80013-241-2 (paperback)
ISBN: 978-1-80013-242-9 (e-book)
ISBN: 978-1-80013-243-6 (PDF)

Typeset by Medlar Publishing Solutions Pvt Ltd, India

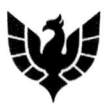

www.firingthemind.com

Contents

Acknowledgements

This book grew up almost naturally from one of our previous joint efforts. Even though we were still intensely focused on our co-edited book on loneliness, it dawned on us that the problem of silencing did not get enough space in our previous book with this word in its very title. We began modestly, but once you start paying attention to silencing, you realise it is everywhere around and inside you.

Being psychoanalysts, we then recognised that something also had to be said about hearing silencing, although (and precisely because) that process is a more mysterious part of therapeutic work. Illustrations were everywhere, from earlier that day or decades ago, from psychoanalytic couches, mental health care institutions, various social groups, literature, the arts …

Because of all this, we feel that this book grew implicitly for decades, and it is impossible to name everyone who deserves to be thanked here. Patients, colleagues, friends in direct communication, and artists, historians of everyday life indirectly, shaped our approach to the phenomena discussed in this book long before we were aware of that.

Still, the book would not have grown to fruition without the crucially important support we received from some individuals in the most recent period:

Kate Pearce supported our project even when we ourselves struggled with its enormous volume and offered advice and patience in her uniquely professional yet heart-warming ways. Everyone else at Karnac worked hard on improving our manuscript, most of all Anita Mason, who caringly supervised all the phases of this manuscript's transformation into a book, and James Darley who brought elegance to our English style.

We benefited greatly from repeated in-depth conversations about our initial ideas with many (old and new) friends. Salman Akhtar, Tobias Blümel, Yael Danieli, Amra Delić, Jay Frankel, Roger Frie, Sue Grand, Gail Hornstein, Vladimir Ivanović, Katerina Kralova, and Lutz Wittmann deserve special mention.

We also thank Ofra Bloch, Peter Fonagy, and Tilman Habermas for kindly agreeing to write blurbs that were so generous.

Aleksandar Dimitrijević would like to thank the Archives and archivists of the University of Essex for the permission to include an entire unpublished letter from Anna Freud to Michael Balint.

Most of all, we appreciate the patience and hard work of our seven contributors, who shared their knowledge and experience by spending many hours focused on these dark issues. We were all guided by the hope that opening these topics is the only way to understand the underlying mechanisms of trauma-related disorders and help victims overcome them. And maybe even more than that.

About the editors and contributors

Editors

Michael B. Buchholz is professor of social psychology at the International Psychoanalytic University (IPU), Berlin (Germany). He is a psychologist and social scientist and a fully trained psychoanalyst. He is head of the doctorate programme at IPU and chair of the social psychology department. He has published more than twenty books and more than 350 scientific papers on topics like the analysis of therapeutic metaphors and therapeutic conversation, including the supervisory process, and he has contributed to psychoanalytic treatment technique, theory, and history. He has conducted conversation analytic studies on group therapy with sexual offenders, about therapeutic "contact scenarios" and on therapeutic empathy. His actual interests are the study of therapeutic talk-in-interaction using conversation analysis. Together with Anssi Peräkylä (Helsinki) he edited a "Frontiers in Psychology" research topic "Talking and Cure—What's Really Going On in Psychotherapy".

Aleksandar Dimitrijević, PhD, is a clinical psychologist and psychoanalyst in private practice in Berlin. He worked as a university lecturer for more than twenty years. He has given lectures, seminars, university courses, and conference presentations throughout Europe and in the US. He is the author of many conceptual and empirical papers about attachment theory and research, psychoanalytic education, and psychoanalysis and the arts, some of which have been translated into German, Hungarian, Italian, Polish, Slovenian, Spanish, and Turkish. He has also edited or co-edited twelve books or special journal issues, the most recent of which are *Ferenczi's Influence on Contemporary Psychoanalytic Traditions* (with Gabriele Cassullo and Jay Frankel), and *Silence and Silencing in Psychoanalysis* and *From the Abyss of Loneliness to the Bliss of Solitude* (both with Michael B. Buchholz).

Contributors

Ana Altaras Dimitrijević, PhD, is a full professor at the Department of Psychology, University of Belgrade. Her teaching and research cover topics from educational and differential psychology, with a special focus on intelligence, giftedness, and meaningful cognitive assessment. From 2010 onwards she has repeatedly served as expert consultant in state-initiated projects on gifted education and has designed and delivered a variety of trainings and workshops for school personnel, to promote differentiated/individualised instruction and inclusive gifted education. Dr Altaras Dimitrijević has authored two books on giftedness (in Serbian: *Giftedness and Underachievement*, 2006; *The Education of High-ability Students: Scientific Foundations and School-practice Guidelines*, 2016), and edited one (*Giftedness: Reflections and Inspections*).

Uta Blohm (born 1967) has studied Lutheran/Reformed Theology in Bochum, Heidelberg, and Wuppertal. She was trained and ordained as a pastor by the Lutheran/Reformed Church in Germany prior to moving to London where her two children were born. Uta has worked for the United Reformed Church in the UK and as a hospital chaplain for the NHS. She has also worked as a hospital chaplain for the Lutheran Church in Hanover (2017–2022).

Uta has been involved in inter-faith dialogue since her student days. Her PhD thesis, "Religious tradition and personal stories. Women working as priests, ministers and rabbis" (2005), deals with issues of inter-faith relations, feminism, and identity.

Uta trained as an integrative psychotherapist at the Minster Centre in London and is currently working in private practice in Hanover. She has been living with her family in Hanover since 2013.

Roger Frie is currently visiting scholar of sociology at CUNY Graduate Center in New York. He is professor of education at Simon Fraser University and affiliate professor of psychiatry at the University of British Columbia in Vancouver, and associate member of the Columbia University Seminar on Cultural Memory and faculty member and supervisor at William Alanson White Institute of Psychiatry, Psychoanalysis and Psychology in New York. He has a private practice in Vancouver and lectures and writes on historical trauma, cultural memory, and moral responsibility related to mass racial violence, genocide, and the Holocaust. He has published numerous books, including the award-winning title, *Not in My Family: German Memory and Responsibility after the Holocaust* (Oxford University Press, 2017). Most recently, he is the editor, with Pascal Sauvayre, of *Culture, Politics and Race in the Making of Interpersonal Psychoanalysis* (Routledge, 2022). His newest book is titled *Edge of Catastrophe: Erich Fromm, Fascism and the Holocaust* (Oxford University Press, 2024). www.rogerfrie.ca

Stephen Frosh has recently retired as professor in the Department of Psychosocial Studies at Birkbeck, University of London. He has a background in academic and clinical psychology and was consultant clinical psychologist and latterly vice dean at the Tavistock Clinic, London, throughout the 1990s. He is a fellow of the Academy of Social Sciences, an academic associate of the British Psychoanalytical Society, a founding member of the Association of Psychosocial Studies, and an honorary member of the Institute of Group Analysis. He is visiting professor at the University of Witwatersrand, South Africa, and at the University of São Paulo, Brazil.

Stephen Frosh is the author of many books and papers on psychosocial studies and on psychoanalysis. His books include

Those Who Come After: Postmemory, Acknowledgement and Forgiveness (2019), *Hauntings: Psychoanalysis and Ghostly Transmissions* (2013), *Psychoanalysis Outside the Clinic* (2010), and *Hate and the Jewish Science* (2005). His most recent book is *Antisemitism and Racism: Ethical Challenges for Psychoanalysis*, published by Bloomsbury in 2023.

Babette Gekeler is a clinical psychotherapist running a transcultural practice, a lecturer at the International Psychoanalytic University of Berlin, and co-director of the Working Group on Refugee and Mental Wellbeing at the Refugee Research Network. Her special research interests lie in the investigation of cultural, racial, and religious belonging and their relation to mental well-being and illness. Further, she is keen on combining her academic rigour and clinical practice to further bridging gaps between science and knowledge development and human lived experience. Participatory methodologies are therefore at the heart of her research engagement and interest. She received her PhD from University College London on public engagement with multiculturalism for which she received a fellowship from the UK's Economic and Social Research Council in 2007. Since 2011 she has had regular engagements as a public speaker on issues relating to identity, group dynamics, and well-being.

Gail A. Hornstein is professor emerita of psychology at Mount Holyoke College, South Hadley, Massachusetts, USA. Her research centres on the contemporary history and practices of psychology, psychiatry, and psychoanalysis, and her articles and opinion pieces have appeared in many scholarly and popular publications. She is author of two books: *To Redeem One Person Is to Redeem the World: The Life of Frieda Fromm-Reichmann* (Other Press, 2005), which questions standard assumptions about treatment through the story of a pioneering psychiatrist, and *Agnes's Jacket: A Psychologist's Search for the Meanings of Madness* (Routledge, 2018), which shows how the insights of people diagnosed with psychosis can challenge fundamental assumptions about mental health, community, and human experience. Her *Bibliography of First-Person Narratives of Madness in English*, now in its fifth edition with more than 1,000 titles, is used internationally by educators, clinicians, and peer organisations. She directs the Hearing Voices Research Project (a national research and training effort in the US, supported by the Foundation for Excellence in Mental Health Care), and speaks widely about mental health issues across the US, UK, and Europe. www.gailhornstein.com

Hans-Christoph Ramm, PhD, born 1949, is a literary and cultural critic. He teaches at the University of the Third Age, Goethe-University, Frankfurt, Germany. He has published on early modern and modern themes: Shakespeare, Dickens, Kafka, V. Woolf, A. Miller, among others.

Introduction: silencing the traumatised and hearing silencing

Aleksandar Dimitrijević and Michael B. Buchholz

Silencing is not a frequent, everyday word in English. In many languages, there are no specific words for this phenomenon (for instance, in German, you have to say "zum Schweigen bringen"—literally "to bring to silence"). While both the professionals and the general public are increasingly aware of the importance of trauma, silencing, which follows trauma almost ubiquitously, remains under the radar. PEP-Web contains only a handful of papers with the word silencing in their titles, which are all very recent—one from 2007 and four published during the last five years. Hopefully, we are slowly waking up.

The prospects are even worse with the phrase "hearing silencing" (which is never mentioned on PEP-Web). One may even wonder what it means and how it is supposed to be done. Like hearing the silence in psychoanalytic sessions and everyday conversions was not tricky enough (see Dimitrijević & Buchholz, 2020b)!? Or hearing the persons silenced by some traumatic experience(s) or relationship(s) during their development finally open up and articulate "their voices" is not challenging enough emotionally!? This book goes one step further as it is an invitation to closely observe the very practices and processes of silencing used by perpetrators of abuse and totalitarian institutions alike.

Both our clinical practices and research endeavours have taught us that silencing is everywhere around us all the time, nowadays, as well as throughout historical epochs. It is essential to remember that trauma gets followed by silence and silencing so often that they can both seem as its integral parts. Also, we could say that it is not possible to overcome trauma because silencing and silence that surround it leave more profound consequences. We must try to understand those processes the best we can to become capable to recognise and prevent their effects.

Moreover, we have embarked on this project of exploring some of the darkest aspects of human communication because we believe that it is actually silencing more than trauma per se that leads to mental pain and disorders. And we want to proclaim that only the acceptance of this and a focus on hearing silencing can finally fulfil psychoanalysis's intersubjective capacity and promise.

In this introduction, we will review, first, conceptual considerations related to silencing and hearing silencing, and then, second, the chapters that build this book.

Silencing and hearing silencing: conceptual considerations

How to recognise silencing?

We need to begin with the question of why silence, sometimes for many years or even a whole lifetime, accompanies trauma. There are different ethical and legal implications to this question, but, viewed from a psychological perspective, the answers are, although complex, in most cases unambiguous. We will here review some of its most significant aspects.

Many traumatised persons go through the process that we call self-silencing. They do not know how to present and explain their experiences and feelings to others and/or themselves. Thus, they carry them in silence, unable to articulate them. Many of them, however, may behave like this for a variety of different reasons:

- The definition of trauma indicates that it is an experience that cannot be integrated with the rest of the personality and is expected to occur in dreams or flashbacks rather than in dialogues;
- Our attention as victims or witnesses is focused on the horrors of suffering and not on the silence and silencing that surround it, and

they do not have to seem as integral parts of what is happening, which leads to their exclusion from sharing with others;

- Children very often grow up accustomed to certain forms of abuse, so they do not think that there is anything to say about it or have not adopted/developed the words through which these painful experiences can be named and expressed;
- Members of groups who have survived social trauma avoid talking about their experiences, hoping that this self-silencing will protect others, especially their children and grandchildren, from the presumed overload.

Silence, of course, can also result from an active effort, conscious or unconscious, to prevent the victim, and sometimes the perpetrator and the witness, from revealing the facts surrounding their trauma(s). In all these situations, we are talking about silencing.

Every group—family, class, company, and state, not to mention "totalitarian institutions" such as churches, prisons, military barracks, monasteries, and psychiatric hospitals—has developed mechanisms for silencing victims. Interestingly, these practices were described first in social science literature under the heading "asylums" (e.g. Foucault, 1975; Goffman, 1961). The perpetrators do not want other people to know, the victims do not want to be perceived as different and labelled, and witnesses do not have the strength to face the pain and fear of punishment. To achieve this, each one resorts to the so-called "conspiracy of silence" (Danieli, 1984), which does not have to be explicitly agreed upon, but all integrated members of one community are aware of the topics that should better be avoided.

The mechanisms by which this is achieved are numerous. Again, listening to and thinking about trauma is difficult, so we can easily deny it with exclamations like "I cannot believe it!", "I'm stunned!", or "Impossible!" Many people, for example, find it unbearable to imagine themselves as a traumatised child, and it is probably impossible to ever fully imagine the loss of a body part or sexual abuse that has never happened to us.

An adult who physically or sexually abuses a child may threaten her that disclosure will lead to an even worse punishment, or try to bribe the child with gifts. Witnesses can deny the possibility ("Don't talk nonsense", "I know him, he would never do it") or minimise its seriousness ("It happens to everyone", "You know how many times I have ...",

"Everyone needs that"), whether they honestly believe in that or are being hypocritical. In some cases of marital violence, the victim may choose to remain silent because of begging and promises, which are, as a rule, not fulfilled later.

In addition, a parent-witness may have been a victim of the same abuser and cannot protect the child because of, for example, fear of retaliation.

People often hope that silence will help traumatised people or at least not remind them of painful experiences, and many victims believe that their problems would burden others and thus try to protect others from themselves by keeping silent. This often happens between parents and children or grandparents and grandchildren, where silence is often seen as a protective shield for the young.

At another level, large groups working to expel, kill, or exterminate entire communities use silencing mechanisms that target many people at once. Over the last hundred years, propaganda has served many times and in many different societies to convince people that they should not believe their eyes or ask any questions. All too often, victims are dehumanised and treated not as persons but as numbers without names, personality traits, and emotions. Through pseudoscientific approaches such as eugenics or typified jokes, members of certain groups are described as less valuable or even as if they do not belong to the human race at all. Witnesses can be subjected to various forms of social pressure, such as discrediting, marginalisation, ostracism, censorship, imprisonment, and assassination.

Some large groups or nations that have committed mass atrocities, war crimes, or genocides barely ever mention the wrongdoings that they did. Change usually has to wait for at least twenty years until a new generation grows up and starts asking questions about guilt from the past. Sometimes one is reminded of the biblical word that the cure of so many cruelties, atrocities, and crimes takes seven generations—and during that time, many other events follow and cover the initial trauma, which makes the artistic expression of collective traumatic experiences essential (see Dimitrijević, 2020).

Throughout history, and in many societies even nowadays, women have been prohibited from access to education, the professions, and financial independence, which is why they could not raise children on their own, and usually cannot return to their parents as divorcees. It was often impossible for them to protect themselves or anyone else, and they had no choice but to suffer in silence.

Many modern humanitarian and social organisations and professions, such as coaching, often claim that it is more important to focus on the future than on the past, on positive thoughts and feelings, so despite possible good intentions, they effectively silence the expression of pain and produce more harm than good.

What are the consequences of silencing?

An experience is traumatic because it is utterly unexpected, uncontrollable, and unpredictable, and it remains difficult to imagine, distance oneself from, and analyse. Worse still, an individual faced with rejection and disbelief almost automatically begins to doubt his or her mind. The younger the victim, the more likely she is to be subjected to "silencing herself". The biggest problem is that a child trusts adults more than herself. Her parents seem to be almost omnipotent, more practically than intellectually. They are disproportionately taller and more robust, so the child also thinks they understand her feelings and motivations better than she can. If, therefore, the adult who has such a role refuses to believe in the testimony about child abuse, the psychological consequences for the child will fall into one or more of these categories:

1. **Splitting.** The most significant number of cases of abuse occurs in family homes, and abusers, in over 90 per cent of cases men, are well known to the child—fathers, grandfathers, uncles, older brothers, family friends, and next-door neighbours. In many of these relationships, the child is attached to the perpetrator, and he initially plays the role of a "secure base" in the child's life, a source of comfort and motivation to explore the physical, social, and mental worlds. Disorders in the child's mind occur because it is impossible to reconcile attachment to, for example, the father and the fact that he is, at the same time, the source of fear and pain. If left alone, the child must maintain a positive mental image of the father and therefore denies, "refuses to believe", that the abuse occurred, even in cases where it is repeated. The process mentioned above creates

a split between the idealised image of the father with which reality is harmonised and the child's perception of her- or himself as terrible, accompanied by a feeling of guilt, an unconscious belief that the child caused everything, and feelings of inadequacy, badness, and worthlessness.

2. **Superficiality in emotional processing.** Especially in preschool age, a child will not survive without her parents but can without her mind, so she renounces her mind when faced with a choice between the two. If my father abuses me, and my mother does not believe me, I begin to think that I invented it all, that I either hallucinated it all or developed it out of malice (the child, of course, would not be able to verbalise it like this). As a result, the capacity for profound emotional processing, commitment to inner mental contents, interest in one's own and others' motives and intentions, and even interest in feelings, closeness, or dreams disappears or never develops (Dimitrijević, 2020; Fonagy et al., 2002), to the extent that some people spend almost their entire lives in loneliness and avoiding others.

3. **Separation of memory, thinking, and feeling functions.** People who suffer from any disorder associated with trauma cannot remember the initial event exactly; they cannot reason, speak coherently about it, and experience the feelings that accompany it (see Allen, 2006). Because of that, for example, memories appear suddenly, in dreams or as "flashbacks", accompanied by intense emotions and physiological reactions, but also by the victim's fear that he will "lose his mind" and that he cannot think about them. Or someone keeps coming back to the same topic, recounting some horrible event in detail, and analysing the details, but at the same time, he is emotionally frozen; the feelings that would be expected to follow the memory are missing.

The combination of trauma and silence/silencing can, therefore, lead to complex personality disorders, addictions, low quality of life, and mental disorders. Many studies conducted in different countries confirm that people diagnosed with mental disorders report many times higher levels of trauma than the general population (see Dimitrijević, 2015). What makes the situation even worse is that many perceive the treatments—especially coercive hospitalisations, electroshocks, and asylums from which there is no hope of ever getting out—as a repeated combination of trauma and silencing.

In contrast, a traumatised child to whom at least one person offers trust, support, and understanding has a high chance of overcoming the problem and even growing into someone who understands someone else's pain better and can offer more help. Almost three quarters of psychotherapists report painful childhood experiences (usually chronic illnesses in the family, most often depressed mothers), with pronounced resilience and the capacity to understand feelings and intentions (Dimitrijević, 2018).

4. **Somatisation.** One of the most apparent consequences of silencing (and/or self-silencing) is the phenomenon of somatisation, considered, among other things, the basis of psychosomatic diseases. Emotions, sensations, and impulses that cannot be mentalized remain or turn into bodily reactions: heart palpitations, skin rashes, asthmatic breathing, incontinence … The same is the case with emotional reactions that are forbidden from expression (and cannot be sublimated, to use Freud's language). For instance, the anger we do not dare express can become a stiff neck. All too often, to hear what was silenced, we have to listen to the body and not to the words.

5. **Social isolation.** A silenced person might develop feelings of worthlessness, badness, inadequacy, shame, and fear that the experience could repeat in social situations. Also, the perpetrator can persuade the victim that this will undoubtedly happen. The victim then chooses rather to stay isolated than share the experience with anyone due to the feeling that social interaction could harm and does not bring anything valuable anyway, although loneliness is one of the most painful experiences for every human being (see Dimitrijević & Buchholz, 2022).

The mechanisms of silencing

If silence leaves such far-reaching consequences, it is essential to understand how this happens. The better we understand the mechanisms/practices of silencing, the better we will be able to develop strategies to prevent its occurrence or eliminate the consequences if it has already occurred. However, not enough is known about this. The number of potential practices at the individual and societal levels, their possible phases, mutual influences, differences concerning age and cultural affiliation—none of this has been systematically and sufficiently investigated yet. What follows is, therefore, a preliminary list.

- **Isolation.** Even without any knowledge of psychoanalysis and psychology, every abuser knows that the most important thing is to isolate the victim before and most often after the abuse. It is easier to beat, insult, rape, and imprison someone if you deny them the support of close persons. That is why the victim is either lured to a secret place or put in conflict with those who might dare to defend her. Especially when it comes to children, the act is a surprise since the perpetrator is usually extraordinarily kind and generous until that moment.

  In many cases of repeated abuse, although not always, the abuser tries to keep the victim in isolation. It is often not a matter of physical isolation but forcing the victim to believe that no one can be trusted. For that, threats, blackmail, and bribery are used, but convincing the victim that no one will believe her anyway, that everyone would laugh at her—and thus, avoid her out of disbelief.

- **Narcissistic seduction.** Many abusers do their best to convince the victim that she was chosen because of her uniqueness and that harassment is the most substantial proof of her uniqueness. The victim is made to believe that only she understands that gods or angels chose her, that it is her unique talent, irresistibility, and capacity to help the abuser and "save" him. The victim should then suffer pain, insults, sexual exploitation, or slavery because they are presented to her as a reward and a sign of mercy. Contrary to all of this, some abusers present themselves as "chosen", as if they know how to or can do something that "mere mortals" will never be able to do. As a rule, they gather followers, make a strict selection, and present abuse as mercy they give to someone. In both cases, the victims are silent because they are afraid they will lose a specialness they are now convinced they have received.

  Many victims also feel that their experience of abuse is unique and that something like that has never happened to anyone else. Because of that, they feel shame, which relates to narcissism, further isolating them because who could confuse others and at the same time admit that she does not deserve respect in her own opinion?

- **Feelings of guilt.** Many victims feel they are to blame for what happened to them, which can be especially noticed in abused children. This is an unconscious mechanism by which the abuser's guilt "ends up" "in" the victim, who begins to recognise it as her own and acts as if she caused everything (Dimitrijević, 2020). When it comes to intense feelings, a child may believe that she is (irreparably) bad and try all her life to help others, save and preserve them, or make everyone happy (Frankel, 2015). The persecutory guilt does not have to be the result of physical or sexual abuse. It can also come from chronic somatic illness or depression in the family that the child thinks he or she caused or from direct parental criticism, demands, and accusations.

- **Identification with the aggressor.** A practice of silencing similar to the previous one can be used in a generalised way. In these cases, the victim may, to a large extent or entirely unconsciously, take the perpetrator's position and feel within herself what she suspects the perpetrator expects from her (Frankel, 2018). (This does not have to include any third person against whom the victim will become aggressive.) Therefore, the victim may feel that she deserves this "punishment" and do whatever she thinks the perpetrator expects in order to forgive and love her again. This process is painfully apparent in people who do not show authenticity; they do not dare to make their own decisions or think independently. Everything we see in them and what they can see in themselves is built to adjust and identify with the aggressor's expectations.

- **Linguistic tools for silencing.** Although it sounds paradoxical, language is a compelling means of silence. It can be used directly or indirectly. An excellent illustration of the direct use is that in Germany, after the Second World War, the word "Nestbeschmutzer" appeared, literally "the one who makes the nest dirty, the nest-polluter". It was a label and a source of pressure for those who refused to remain silent about the crimes committed during Nazism. Implicitly, it also included a claim that the nest (homeland and individual family homes) was clean (without guilt) as long as everyone remained silent. A prevalent version of this is telltale, a word used derogatorily even when a child wants to report peer violence. Indirect use refers to the fact that some words or expressions necessary for expression or accusation are not something we learn spontaneously at home or as a part of instruction at school. After a certain number of sessions, many psychotherapeutic patients try to talk about the abuse for the first time but do not know the right words. The problem is not only euphemisms (for example, "educational slaps" as a description of physical abuse in schools) but the fact that talking and listening about trauma is usually avoided and that the terminology for its definition is not developed. It is enough to remember the silence surrounding sexuality—how parents rarely initiate conversations with children, interrupt their questions, or change television channels.

- **Denial of the right to education.** The primary mechanism of abuse of women for thousands of years has not been physical force or weapons but the rejection of the girls' right to attend schools, become literate, and choose professions. Most women are financially dependent and cannot leave the perpetrator. In patriarchal societies, parents will not accept them as divorcees, and they cannot support themselves and their children. Another critical aspect of girls' education is not being introduced to basic knowledge about conception, pregnancy, and contraception. A woman who has her profession and source of income and can decide and control how many children she will have can hardly be subjugated and turned into an enslaved person.

  In many societies, especially where monotheistic religions play a crucial role, the same is true for boys, that is, men. The translation of the Bible into the languages that people use in everyday life, for which some were burned at stakes in London in the sixteenth century, is a consequence of the insight that it is easier to rule over illiterate and dependent people. An updated instance is the attempt to murder Malala Yousafzai, who in 2012 was shot in the head point-blank by a Pakistani Taliban for advocating that girls should be allowed access to education.

- **Centralisation of power.** Every dictatorship strives to establish a system where all decisions will be made in one place or even by one person. The space for discussion, consideration of various possibilities, voting, and the opposition's existence are abolished. In the ideological domain, only one voice remains, and everything else is silenced. Although formally there may be institutions and divisions into, say, republics, regions, and municipalities, all decisions come from the same place as none of the people who work there dare to express their opinion or take any initiative. Leaders of the Nazi party believed they were capable of classifying art, Stalin also "knew" how to compose and write novels, and Tito gave speeches against jazz. It is unusual but repeatedly confirmed that huge masses are willing to remain silent for decades and, over time, lose the capacity to make decisions; they become dependent, like the citizens of many colonised countries, just as sociologists describe adult patients in psychiatric asylums (e.g. Goffman, 1961).

- **Propaganda and censorship.** Political organisations, specific ideological orientations, and interest groups, such as financial ones, use the mass media and even the educational process to convince all the users that only their ideas are correct and only their products are valuable. This was widely used by Josef Goebbels, Hitler's minister of propaganda, and in Soviet cinematography and arts, and has in recent decades become the primary purpose of countless television channels, which bombard their audiences with advertising without ever double-checking the actual quality of consumer products or political figures and organisations. And such is the enormity of this trend, now also on social media, that one is constantly, probably in all countries and languages, flooded by propaganda to the level that truth can quickly be silenced as just one among millions of voices.

During this process, all other voices—political or commercial competition—are either squeezed out with the hope that no one will hear of them or belittled and portrayed as less valuable or dangerous. Thus, in totalitarian regimes, only one voice can remain in the political arena. However, such fear creeps into citizens that they are no longer allowed to talk about the traumas they are experiencing on their own, either on a social-collective or individual level. In regimes called democratic, on the other hand, such a large number of voices is often heard that none of them matters anymore (for example, in the form of the "right" to have and express an opinion on topics about which one knows nothing), or the voices change at such a tempo that they become irrelevant after a few days. Such efforts could be directly focused on banning the publication of information on mass crimes (in the Soviet Union, for example, it was not allowed to write about Nazi pogroms against Jews in Ukraine), convincing the public that a crime did not happen or that it was an accidental consequence of good intent (like the regular depiction of the colonisation of Africa, the Americas, Australia, and India), but they are also about powerful companies persuading us that their latest products will solve all our problems, or well-connected managers presenting their latest client as the most talented musician ever. It is regrettable for us as psychoanalysts that this whole field was grounded in his books by Freud's nephew, Edward Bernays, the so-called father of public relations.

- **Dehumanisation.** Victims are often portrayed as less valuable or unworthy of being included in the human race, so crimes against them are committed without a bad conscience, at least on a conscious level. Thus, the Nazis reduced all their victims to numbers, without name and surname, origin, age, education, marital status, and social status, as expressed in income and dressing like a hobo or tramp, losing all rights to use administrative support or public transportation. So every day, they killed certain number-bearers, calling them lice, with whom it was impossible to sympathise. During the war in Bosnia and Herzegovina, similar (eugenic) views were spread, claiming that Bosnian Muslims were carriers of bad genes because their ancestors changed religion out of weakness and killing them was simply cleansing society of an irreparably inferior group, otherwise previously marked by jokes always presenting them as hopelessly stupid. The worst part of this process is that the victims accept the hatred of others towards themselves and the feeling of worthlessness and deserving punishment, and thus the belief that it makes no sense to complain and express their suffering.

- **Conspiracy of silence.** Large groups sometimes do not mention a crime for years or decades, although no explicit agreement has been reached (see Danieli, 1984). Everyone is silent about it; it is not in newspapers or books, children do not learn about it in history classes, and families and friends do not discuss it. Once it is discovered what actually happened, no one can explain how the conspiracy of silence came about or who initiated it. On the level of smaller groups, the conspiracy of silence can be a matter of convenience, comfort, profit, family dynamics, and the structure of mafia organisations.

As mentioned, those who try to break this conspiracy are often threatened, labelled, or ostracised, so this is likely kept intact due to fear, isolation, and other mechanisms listed here. One excellent illustration for this is *Afterward*, a documentary by Dr Ofra Bloch, a psychoanalyst and filmmaker from New York, who tried to radically listen to those she was raised to regard as the other—the Germans and the Palestinians—and occupy her double role as victim and perpetrator. Her efforts to make sense of the present and open the door for a future—an afterward—were met with acts of silencing from various groups, which aimed to discard any narrative not based on the schematic and oversimplified binary of us/them and victims/perpetrators.

How to hear silencing?

The history of psychoanalysis is full of evolving steps of listening. Initially, it was named a "talking cure" by Bertha Pappenheim, a patient of Josef Breuer. Then, Freud taught a whole culture how to listen to "slips" and read or listen to unconscious intentions. Theodor Reik (1948) coined the term "listening with the third ear". Another line of thinking about listening was opened when Haydée Faimberg (1996) taught us vertical steps, like "listening to listening". Others joined with the observation that we "see" images while we "hear" words. Musical listening in the treatment room could be described and connected (see Grassi, 2021) with evolving skills of talk and formulation. Donnel B. Stern (2009) made an enormous step forward when he guided clinicians' attention to the ways of hearing unformulated experiences. The multiple variations of silence became an object of study, and silence could no longer be considered the opposite of talking but an element of it (Dimitrijević & Buchholz, 2020). And, because we must breathe in and breathe out, we learned to view silences as an embodied rhythmic structuring of our talk. We follow this historical line of evolving clinical skills in understanding silencing and responding to it.

This book is guided by the idea that there is not only silence but robust silencing processes—directed to others and oneself. Silencing—this is an unusual word; it points to "being made silent", following a powerful imperative of "Don't tell!", "Never talk about"—and creates a clinical and theoretical challenge. How can we think of elementary life events never shared with anybody else? How can a therapist ever get the hunch of an idea that there is something to be told about which the potential teller still has no grasp? Is this an unconscious process or unconscious "material"?

The answer our contributors here point at is that silencing is the malignant consequence of power—and we immediately come to see that "power" is a human dimension, which still has not attracted much theoretical attention and energy in psychoanalysis. Power is, as it were, a silenced topic in the history of psychoanalysis, too. Being silenced is an intrinsic aspect of being traumatised, and psychoanalysis is not free from this in its history. Being silenced is also a social topic, and it all depends on the human capacity for listening, receptivity, and endurance.

The problem of silencing is so sinister and ubiquitous simultaneously that attempts to open closed mouths would have to be systematic and well organised. Here is a sketch of the many levels of these attempts, all based on the general assumption derived from clinical practice that "change needs connection" (Buchholz, 2019).

1. **Trauma-focused psychotherapy.** Both individuals and small groups who experience trauma and do not get the opportunity to express their pain need access to effective forms of psychotherapy. It should not be forgotten that the term "talking cure" was first used by one patient to let her doctor know that nothing helped her as much as the opportunity to talk about everything that was coming to her mind and thus completely overcome all forms of silencing that she was exposed to. Almost a century and a half has passed since then, and various psychotherapeutic approaches have been developed, many of which have been empirically confirmed to be helpful. In addition to the further development of psychotherapy, which is necessary, it is crucial to make these achievements available to as many victims as possible. This specifically means that it is required to:

   - Train many professionals to be able to listen to traumatic experiences and help those who have experienced them
   - Decentralise mental health services so that (among other things) psychotherapy becomes available throughout each country

- Make psychotherapy available free of charge for persons suffering from certain mental disorders through the state's financial support for specific institutions
- "Detoxify" psychotherapists' programmes to intervene "against" symptoms or develop programmes for (or against) silencing; "just listen" is a better device; to quote prominent researchers, introduce psychotherapy as a "low-level technology" (Wampold & Imel, 2015), after a most thorough worldwide overview of psychotherapy outcome research.

2. **Psychological support to families.** Throughout their development, which lasts several decades, families are fragile systems facing numerous challenges. This refers to the skills of overcoming (inevitable) conflicts without the use of (physical) force, ways to recognise children's needs and support their independence, finding new purpose in the "empty nest", and discovering the meaning of old age. Parents need to recognise the signs of trauma or depression in their children, ways to help themselves, and when and how to turn to professional help. In many marriages, it is necessary to accept the idea of equality, whether it is in decision-making, financial plans, or sex life. In every family, it is necessary to develop the habit of talking openly about feelings, problems, and fears of feeling silenced.

3. **Literacy.** Mass literacy still needs to be achieved in many countries of South-Eastern Europe and on many other continents. People must have a sense of independence, a professional identity, access to essential information, and feel enough self-esteem to defend their dignity.

   In recent years, the process of "emotional literacy", helping people acquire basic skills of recognising feelings in themselves and others, and expressing, naming, and discussing them, has been mentioned more and more often. These processes are most probably closely related to the increasing use of the internet, smartphones, and social networks since the "dictionary of feelings" is learned from literature, especially poetry, in which there is less and less interest among younger generations.

4. **Education to respect others.** All institutions, from the family to the national assembly, governments, and courts, have the opportunity to treat other persons as equal subjects, with respect for their integrity

and dignity, or to direct all their power to subjugate and enslave them. The educational process must include a focus on understanding the importance of human rights, protection, and respect, both in the political and private spheres. This could, over time, reduce the occurrence of abuse (many forms of which are still not recognised as abuse today), as well as the silencing of anyone's voice.

5. **Art education.** Psychological research shows that this is most easily achieved through a focus on artistic expression in school education. If you want children to be more empathetic, empathise more and more accurately, and be more willing to help others, introduce them to as many hours of singing, drawing, songwriting, or drama sessions as possible (Winner & Hetland, 2008). This requires expressing certain feelings, imagining other persons' feelings, as in a character in the play, or someone else who drew something, which will later be transferred to everyday life.

6. **Change and consistent application of the laws.** It is necessary to change many existing laws and adopt many new ones to establish independent human rights institutions consistently. All victims of individual or social trauma should be provided with psychological support and legal protection so that they can feel safeguarded before they dare talk about their experiences. It is true that some of these laws and institutions already exist in some countries. However, it is necessary 1) to insist on the consistent application of these laws, penal policy, and internal control of the police, and 2) to defend their independence from the executive power that longs for it to be the only authority. In the Netherlands, protectors of the rights of psychiatric patients are lawyers employed by an institution independent of both the Ministry of Justice and the Ministry of Health. It is impossible to influence them when, upon patient complaints, they visit mental health institutions and write reports, recommendations, and penalties. In contrast, Serbian protectors of the rights of psychiatric patients are lawyers employed by psychiatric hospitals, whom the directors of those hospitals can fire.

7. **Democratic institutions.** Citizens follow examples from state institutions, from the highest levels to local ones. And just as initiatives are needed that come from mass groups of citizens who protect and demand their rights, it is essential that those in charge set an example

of openness to listening to others, acknowledging and correcting mistakes, respecting limitations, and fulfilling obligations. This is important at the level of everyday events but also when it comes to historical misconceptions and hostilities. All minorities and languages, and a variety of political options, deserve the opportunity to articulate themselves. Democracy is a demanding and slow dialogue, but it is the system that is the least silencing one of all we have tried so far, especially in participatory forms, such as the Swiss one.

We also propose including ethics in therapeutic reasoning as the most relevant dimension in psychotherapy and as the most vital impulse to influence societal institutions.

What is in this book?

Naturally, it is only possible to cover some of the above-mentioned topics in one book. Our effort was focused on what we see as the first step in tackling this challenging topic. In twelve chapters, we provide detailed descriptions of silencing in various contexts and with frighteningly omnipresent influence.

This volume starts with a comprehensive review of the silencing of victims and perpetrators. Forced to silence himself because people refused to hold their ears accessible for him and his survival in Auschwitz, Primo Levi broke down—that no one was open to listening to what he had gone through destroyed his belief in humanity and a common future worth the effort. But he and his fate are only the starting point for an endless series of human beings who endured enormous suffering but could have recovered if only there were someone capable of listening. More than the trauma itself, it is the experience of not finding anybody capable of listening patiently, with warmth and devotion, which destroys the ability to tell one's story and the belief in human sharing.

This lesson runs through the centuries with a clear trace. However, although clearly articulated, it is silenced often enough, even too often. In psychoanalytic training, people are taught a lot of theory and theoretical understanding. Even so, the ability to let oneself become seized is taught only in some supervisory courses (Buchholz, 2015;

Jefferson, 2017). Often enough, theoretical debates prevail; they dominate and silence participation, compassion, and untold experience—not infrequently by ascribing a unique role to "emotions" and ignoring that emotions are consequences of experiences, not their causes (Feldman-Barrett, 2017).

There are many efforts to silence victims, witnesses, and perpetrators. However, fortunately enough, there is the phenomenon of whispering. Certain documents were not burnt, places were not destroyed, and undetected witnesses were not killed. Something or someone survives and, often enough, after decades of silence, begins to whisper, meeting other whisperers, and the whole story emerges like a river starting from the most miniature fountain. All these phenomena can be noticed, observed, and documented by historians and other scientists (e.g. Figes, 2008), and we have the task of reintegrating this into our corpus of clinical and general human knowledge. These efforts sometimes require courage, as clinical institutions have participated, and sometimes still do, in silencing what their clients had to say. It could be a task for the future to clear psychoanalytic theorising from misguided efforts of that kind.

Such efforts could have the potential of hearing Hamlet silencing himself and realising those efforts in the Hamlets of our days. As is shown in the second chapter here, *Hamlet* paradigmatically sensitises careful readers and spectators of human stages to the painful potential of being silenced or silencing oneself. Other pieces, like Grossman's novel *Stalingrad* or Philip Roth's *The Human Stain*, are read here as modern reconfigurations of Hamlet's fate: massive efforts at self-silencing.

Stephen Frosh, in his contribution, points directly to the difference. It is not silence that is addressed here but the acts of silencing happening in institutions established to help traumatised and sexually abused children. Frosh uses the term "murmuring", which comes very close to "whispering", a term which we took from the historian Orlando Figes (2008). The closeness of these two metaphors points to a similar observation of the same event structure; one is a macro perspective of a whole society, Stalin's Russia, and the other is an institution of help and care. And Frosh describes as highly relevant the role of the "second adult", the person who knows and silences what could be observed in cases of child sexual abuse. There is a mode of traumatic identification where observers act as if they were traumatised themselves—they foresee the many serious difficulties, the imposition of personal strength expected from them, and that they must decide which side to take. This decision guides their idea and agenda of help.

Roger Frie, historian, social philosopher, and psychoanalyst, has chosen his topic after a deeply personal exploration of his family's involvement in the times of German National Socialism. This personal "working through" enabled him to write an impressive contribution about the Elaine Massacre in Arkansas in 1919. Anywhere from several hundred to almost a thousand African Americans were shot by white farmers and soldiers. Frie met people whose parents or grandparents had survived. He addressed them as victims in the expectation that they would want to share and make public what they knew from the family conversations. But he found that an event with so many people being killed is incompletely documented by the administration, and people hesitated to talk about what parents and grandparents had told them about it. Whether to continue silence, to murmur or whisper, or to fully share their knowledge depends on a reflection about one's future state in their community; they have to anticipate the effects of talking and sharing concerning what Frie calls the "silence of white complicity". An actual relational context co-determines if something is told or if self-silencing continues.

To talk or remain silent—this is hard to decide also for women who were victims of sexual violence. This is so powerful a fact that Babette S. Gekeler opens her contribution by pointing out the consequences this has for published statistics about the frequency of such events. Silencing controls data. Her reference point is the debate about the US Supreme Court's decision on abortion rights of June 2022. This topic risks the violation of superordinate values as basic guarantees for individual existence. Thus, we cannot question individual rights or possessive individualism, as all human beings have the right to live a life on one's own. People have the right to have rights guaranteeing life on their own, including the right to pursue happiness. Female bodies, in whole or in part, are not in another person's possession, and they are not equivalents of enslaved people. Gekeler speaks of the "silencing of women" with the implicit question of how men position themselves. Why is that? Because men are attracted by female bodies and are abrasively appalled by female bodies. This paradox leaves most men speechless, as the author shows us in a well-informed walk through the history of medicine from Hippocrates to the Middle Ages, including horrible pandemic times and many surprising books from the days when dead female bodies were surgically opened for the first time. Freud can be included in the line of this history, and his way of silencing evidence about some horrible practices in the Vienna of his days has been laid open by Carlo Bonomi, an Italian psychoanalyst on whose work Gekeler draws. Freud was not only a great discoverer. He was a silencer, too.

In the sixth contribution to this book, we describe how another heretic, named "Bento", from the Spinoza family, was silenced in the seventeenth century. All the Amsterdam Jewish community members were forbidden to exchange a single word with him—he had asked too many questions, pointed out inconsistencies in Jewish belief systems, and spent his life writing (and then grinding lenses for eyeglasses and telescopes). It is as if the power of the Inquisition, whose tortures forced many poor people to speak unbelievable truths, is of mighty influence still today but replaced by other silencing forces. Galilei and Copernicus suffered from the same fate, and it is no pleasure to remind psychoanalytic readers that Ernest Jones, Freud's hagiographic biographer, blocked the publication of some of Ferenczi's writings for more than fifty years. But, of course, he claimed, it was in the best interests of Ferenczi's reputation. In this chapter, we are taken through a long history of mutual silencing in and between Jewish and Christian traditions, which is a forerunner for some silencing practices in psychoanalysis.

The next chapter is devoted to another instance of silencing that affects large groups of people, specifically children. Ana Altaras Dimitrijević writes about the destiny of schoolchildren, especially the gifted ones, who are told not to pose questions or solve tasks in their way. Illustrations from three continents make the text convincing, and psychological considerations, like the "stigma of giftedness" or "anti-achievement peer pressure", make it alarming.

From here, we go to the chapter on censorship, which gives an impression of a particular case subsumed under the category of silencing giftedness. This time, it is about ideological control and stifling the voices of creative, sometimes genius artists. From various examples, almost all of which come from the twentieth century, we learn about the power of propaganda and the greed of the powerful to control everything, even the imagination. If we want you to use our symbols, buy our products, express our emotions, and think our thoughts, we have to make everyone sing in unison and eliminate each dissonant voice.

The final third of the book is more directly focused on clinical issues. First, we try to clean our own backyard and discuss the problem of silencing in psychoanalytic institutions. Thanks to the increasing availability of the original documents that were never planned for publication (like correspondence, diaries, minutes), we now know a great deal about various attempts at censoring psychoanalytic publications, ostracising creative members, and, consequently, building institutions on the principles of loyalty and obedience. The subsequent brain drain (also discussed in the chapter) cannot come as a surprise after all this.

Silencing is a ubiquitous clinical phenomenon. We therefore proceed with various illustrations of this, both in the narratives of clients or in the "interventions" of psychotherapists. And once you start paying attention, it becomes evident that every client's traumatic experience is followed by pressure to remain silent. Family therapy seems to be an even more powerful X-ray for detecting these processes than individual treatments. Michael B. Buchholz, this time from the role of a seasoned family therapist, supervisor, and educator, describes situations when several family members can be led to the recognition that current symptoms stem from unexpressed, very often silenced, old pain. The book's finale was focused on a special topic and entrusted to a unique author. Gail Hornstein writes about the silencing of persons with mental disorders, who were (and at many places still are) never asked, quoted, or even named. Hornstein, who has devoted significant portions of her professional career to studying this silencing process and the ways of overcoming it, also describes how she has repeatedly been discouraged from doing research in this domain.

We are delighted that this book has been a medium for all these authors to articulate their perspectives on some of humanity's darkest sides. We hope that the reader(s) will boldly join us in this attempt to hear the unspoken horrors, as that may be the only way to overcome current and prevent future trauma, silencing, and mental disorders.

References

Allen, J. G. (2006). *Traumatic Relationships and Serious Mental Disorders.* Hoboken, NJ: John Wiley & Sons.

Buchholz, M. B. (2015). Listening to words, seeing images—metaphors of emotional involvement and the movement of the metaphor. *Psychoanalytic Discourse, 5*(1): 20–38.

Buchholz, M. B. (2019). Veränderung braucht Verbindung. In: E.-M. Graf, C. Scarvaglieri, & T. Spranz-Fogasy (Eds.), *Pragmatik der Veränderung—Problem- und lösungsorientierte Kommunikation in helfenden Berufen* (pp. 75–95). Berlin: Springer.

Danieli, Y. (1984). Psychotherapists' participation in the conspiracy of silence about the Holocaust. *Psychoanalytic Psychology, 1*(1): 23–42.

Dimitrijević, A. (2015). Trauma as a neglected etiological factor of mental disorders. *Sociologija, 57*(2): 286–299.

Dimitrijević, A. (2018). Why devote your life to psychoanalysis—an impossible profession? Presented at the Chicago Psychoanalytic Society, June 18, 2018.

Dimitrijević, A. (2020). Silence and silencing of the traumatized. In: A. Dimitrijević & M. B. Buchholz (Eds.), *Silence and Silencing in Psychoanalysis. Cultural, Clinical, and Research Perspectives* (pp. 198–216). London: Routledge.

Dimitrijević, A., & Buchholz, M. B. (Eds.) (2020). *Silence and Silencing in Psychoanalysis: Cultural, Clinical, and Research Perspectives.* London: Routledge.

Dimitrijević, A., & Buchholz, M. B. (2022). *From the Abyss of Loneliness to the Bliss of Solitude: Cultural, Social and Psychoanalytic Perspectives.* Bicester, UK: Phoenix.

Faimberg, H. (1996). Listening to listening. *International Journal of Psychoanalysis, 77*: 667–677.

Feldman-Barrett, L. (2017). *How Emotions are Made: The Secret Life of the Brain.* Boston, MA: Houghton Mifflin Harcourt.

Figes, O. (2008). *The Whisperers: Private Life in Stalin's Russia.* London: Penguin.

Fonagy, P., Gergely, G., Jurist, E. L., & Target, M. (2002). *Affect Regulation, Mentalization, and the Development of the Self.* New York: Other Press.

Foucault, M. (1975). *Discipline and Punish: The Birth of the Prison.* A. Sheridan (Trans.). London: Vintage, 1991.

Frankel, J. (2015). The persistent sense of being bad: The moral dimension of identification with the aggressor. In: A. Harris & S. Kuchuck (Eds.), *The Legacy of Sándor Ferenczi: From Ghost to Ancestor* (pp. 204–222). London: Routledge.

Frankel, J. (2018). Psychological enslavement through identification with the aggressor. In: A. Dimitrijević, G. Cassullo, & J. Frankel (Eds.), *Ferenczi's Influence on Contemporary Psychoanalytic Traditions* (pp. 134–139). London: Routledge.

Goffman, E. (1961). *Asylums: Essays on the Social Situation of Mental Patients and Other Inmates.* Garden City, NY: Doubleday.

Grassi, L. (2021). *The Sound of the Unconscious: Psychoanalysis as Music.* Routledge.

Jefferson, G. (2017). *Repairing the Broken Surface of Talk: Managing Problems in Speaking, Hearing, and Understanding in Conversation.* J. R. Bergmann & P. Drew (Eds.). Oxford: Oxford University Press.

Reik, T. (1948). *Listening with the Third Ear: The Inner Experience of a Psychoanalyst.* New York: Farrar, Straus and Giroux.

Stern, D. B. (2009). *Partners in Thought: Working with Unformulated Experience, Dissociation, and Enactment.* New York: Routledge.

Wampold, B. E., & Imel, Z. E. (2015). *The Great Psychotherapy Debate: The Evidence for What Makes Psychotherapy Work.* New York: Routledge.

Winner, E., & Hetland, L. (2008). Art for our sake: School arts classes matter more than ever—but not for the reasons you think. *Arts Education Policy Review, 109*(5): 29–32.

CHAPTER 1

Silencing victims, witnesses, and perpetrators

Michael B. Buchholz, Aleksandar Dimitrijević, and Hans-Christoph Ramm

Introduction

There was a time when intrepid researchers had to report the "conspiracy of silence" even in helping professions, including among psychoanalysts (Danieli, 1984; see also Dimitrijević & Buchholz, 2020). They knew and did not know (Grand, 2013; Jack & Ali, 2010). We encounter this phenomenon almost everywhere and on all the levels of every society. In this chapter, we will focus on the very openly violent aspect of silencing: how victims get silenced by perpetrators and/or witnesses and how witnesses and perpetrators get silenced themselves.

Silencing the victims

The scope—from societal to individual

Many survivors of the Shoah were shattered when they tried to tell other people about their experiences after the war. Primo Levi was devastated by the response of his audience. After his lectures in Munich, many people came up to him, ignorantly patting him on the back and telling him he should be glad to have survived. In the words of a psychoanalyst

1

interned in Buchenwald: "People did not really want me to talk about my experiences, and whenever I started, they invariably showed their resistance by interrupting me, by asking me to tell them how I got out." There were no ears open to hear silencing. As Ellie Wiesel wrote:

> Had we started to speak, we would have found it impossible to stop. Having shed one tear, we would have drowned the human heart. So invincible in the face of death and the enemy, we now felt helpless … we were mad with disbelief. People refused to listen, to understand, to share. There was a division between us and them, between those who endured and those who read about it or would refuse to read about it … we thought people would remember our experiences, and our testimony, and manage to suppress their violent impulses to kill or to hate.[1]

Although the scale is entirely different, this is an experience similar to what raped or physically abused women report about how the police sometimes treat them. Speaking requires receptive ears, or it is silenced again. Non-receptivity to a traumatic experience is possibly worse than the trauma (Dimitrijević, 2020). Hearing silencing is required far beyond the treatment room.

We found a report about the fate of Margarita Gratschewa, a Russian woman who had two children with her ex-husband (Pröll, 2022). She was divorced and lived in a suburb, so her husband had to pick her up every morning in his car—she could not afford one—to bring their children to kindergarten. One morning, he unexpectedly turned off the route, drove into the forest and chopped off both of her hands. Then he brought her to a hospital where one hand was saved surgically.

Some of the details are very illustrative. The day before, she had informed her colleagues that if she was not on time for work the following day, they should inform the police. Indeed, when she failed to show up for work, colleagues took this seriously and did inform the police. But the police did not go looking for her. Her concern was silenced.

However, it is one of the well-known examples where in hindsight, it turns out that victims have predicted acts of violence. Alarm calls

---

[1] Both of these quotes were given after Mucci, 2013, p. 141.

are overheard often enough because they are somewhat encoded. Sometimes, witnesses later remember slightly ambiguous statements, which predict what happened—a pervasive experience of hearing silencing. Many recognise someone's announced suicide in hidden messages. Psychotherapists engaged in supporting husband-beaten women report that these women often cannot *name* the violence or, worse still, even *recognise* it. Also, violence is often romanticised: "If he beats you, he loves you" is a widespread proverb. In some countries, the criminalisation of domestic violence has been suspended. In Russia, this has been the case since 1991, and the EU judges in Strasbourg ruled in December 2021 that the state had to pay Gratchewa €350,000 for failing to pass a law that would have protected her.

A prototype—Ovid

Silencing someone by threats is risky for a perpetrator—maybe the mouth will open to witness the deed after all. Therefore, another form of silencing victims has developed long ago: ripping or cutting out one's tongue. The prototypical literary model for this can be found in Ovid. The unfortunate Philomela's fate was cruel.

> Once Philomel was on the painted ship/ And the oars struck and thrust the land away, / "I've won!" he cried, "I've won! My dearest wish / Is mine on board with me!" His heart leapt high …. / The captive has no chance / Of flight, the captor gloats over his prize. … / And then the king drags off Pandion's daughter / Up to a cabin in the woods, remote / And hidden away among dark ancient trees, / And there pale, trembling, fearing everything, / Weeping and asking where her sister was, / He locked her, and revealed his own black heart / And ravished her, a virgin, all alone, / Calling and calling to her father, calling to / Her sister, calling, even more, to heaven above. / She shivered like a little frightened lamb, / Mauled by a grizzled wolf and cast aside, / And still unable to believe it's safe; / Or as a dove, with feathers dripping blood, / Still shudders in its fear, still dreads the claws, / The eager claws that clutched it. In a while, / When sense returned, she tore her tumbled hair, / And like a mourner

bruised her arms, and cried / With outstretched hands, "You brute! You cruel brute! / Do you care nothing for the charge, the tears / Of my dear father, for my sister's love, / For my virginity, your marriage vows? ... / I'll shed my shame / And shout what you have done. If I've the chance," ... / Goaded by both, that brutal despot drew / His dangling sword and seized her by the hair, / And forced her arms behind her back and bound / Them fast; and Philomela, seeing the sword, / Offered her throat and hoped she would have died. / But as she fought, outraged, for words and called / Her father's name continually, he seized / Her tongue with tongs and, with his brutal sword, / Cut it away. The root jerked to, and fro; / The tongue lay on the dark soil muttering ... / Even after that dire deed / Men say (could I believe it), lusting still, / Often on the poor maimed girl he worked his will. (Ovid, Book 6, lines 422 ff., 1986, pp. 134–142)

Once again, the forest is the place of horror. Both are driving, Gratschewa and her divorced husband in a car, Philomela, and her fiancé Tereus on a boat. Tereus, full of anticipation, exclaims that he has won the most important treasure on board! It looks like a pleasure trip. Then it turns infinitely cruel, and he rapes her. She screams for help. She threatens that even though help will come later she will say all. This warns him. Brutally, he cuts out her tongue. Now she can no longer bear witness. Her silence is her unavoidable destiny. When she reaches her family, she helps herself by writing down the description of what happened. But not many were (or still are) literate.

Philomela's fate was taken up by Shakespeare, who in *Titus Andronicus* shows Lavinia turning the pages of her Ovid in an attempt to detect differences and parallels between her fate and that of Philomela.

In the same *Titus*, another scene illustrates what Shakespeare had learned from Ovid. Ravished and abused as Philomela was, Lavinia cannot even sing when Marcus compares her to Orpheus—she has lost her tongue, too, and, to make matters worse, both her hands were cut off, and she could no longer even write. Again, there are no witnesses to these crimes, and the capacity of the victims to provide testimonies is destroyed.

Psychoanalysts might be inclined to recognise the power of myth here. Instead, we propose to analyse the logic of situations. This logic here is recognisable to the perpetrator because he has to silence the victim/witness. If something of his horrific deed can reach the ears of others, he would be condemned, punished, expelled, tortured, and killed—and these powerful corporal punishments, in turn, have the powerful gestalt logic of deterring possible revenge.

The perfect crime is not only killing the victim but guaranteeing the silence of all witnesses. As court proceedings in totalitarian states often document, this includes the judges. They are silent about what they know, as they have been instructed or, better said, threatened. If no one can witness the crime, the victims are deterred from making statements, and no valid evidence is available, communication is silenced by extracted tongues or other means, then the crime did not even occur. Silencing has won.

Whispering

Silencing often focuses on wiping out words, ripping out tongues, and controlling free speech. Indeed, many people who tried to speak were hindered in their professional advancement, academic careers were blocked, and others were taken to penal camps. These were measures by the sources of political power, making talking impossible or forced into a whisper. Whispering is different from being bowed down. It is an attempt to tell the truth without betraying oneself, which makes one walk upright and proud. Many traumatised people who find nobody to speak with start whispering prayers silently and use an ancient cultural practice to murmur prayers, to whisper to God, and to whisper to one-self (McAffee, 2016). Even though no human being is willingly available to listen, complete silencing is not achieved as you can turn to religious beliefs. However, there are experiences of married couples (Figes, 2008), who only with the political thaw of the 1990s dared confess to each other that they stemmed from bourgeois families, their parents and grandparents were sentenced to many years in Siberia, and the couple managed to hide their true life from each other as deeply as possible. Even a whisper was a high risk.

Even a person like the leader of Perestroika, Mikhail Gorbachev, did not dare to give any insight into his biography until 1990. When he was born in 1931 into a peasant family, his grandfather was sent into exile in Siberia because he was accused of not having harvested enough. That was in the year of the famine, 1933. Gorbachev's maternal grandfather was arrested as a "Trotskyist" in 1937. For a long time, Gorbachev considered this biography "tainted with flaws".

Silencing witnesses

The next element of situational gestalt is the strong pressure to silence the witnesses of certain crimes. As it was recently written,

> The perfect crime, as Jean François Lyotard (1988) claimed, does not consist of killing the victim but rather of obtaining the silence of the witness, the deafness of the judges and the inconsistency of the testimony. If one neutralizes the addressor, the addressee and the significance of the testimony, the result is that there is no referent: no crime has been committed (Lyotard, 1988). This erasure of the referent is achieved by the emergence of a double language, marked by a dissociation between its explicit and its implicit meaning. (Amir & HaCohen, 2020, pp. 297–298)

We will discuss several examples of this.

Erdogan

By the end of January 2022, several newspapers reported a new step in Turkey's cultural fight. These were initiated by President Erdogan, who annulled the law which protected women against male violence. Now, men's attacks on women are prosecuted less frequently, if at all. The situation is the worst for married women, who can be beaten or attacked in other ways by their husbands, who are set free from prosecution. On January 25, Erdogan publicly verbally attacked three women, two of them, Sezen Akzu and Sedef Kabas, prominent musicians of Turkish pop. In their public announcements on social media, both quoted a proverb: "If an ox goes to a palace, he does not become a king. The palace becomes a stable." Erdogan's campaign against the singers started with the suppression of free speech and turned to misogyny. The government suddenly discovered that a song by Sezen Akzu, which was in the charts for more than five years, offended religious feelings. The singer positions herself politically with her song on "the ignorant Adam and Eve". In Islam, Adam is a prophet. Thus, disrespect is not allowed. Erdogan, after prayers in the Istanbul Camlica mosque, cried: "Nobody is entitled to insult the prophet, Adam!" And added: "Should anyone do so, it is our duty to rip out their tongue." Akzu's friends, artists, other singers showed broad solidarity and published warningly: nobody is safe.

Katyn

In April 1940, after Germany had attacked Poland from the West and the Soviet Union attacked Poland from the East, Stalin's secret service NKVD executed more than 14,500 Polish military officers and more than 7,000 civilians. The place of the massacre was Katyn, a hidden forest in the Polish East. It took a long time to establish the historical facts. All those involved tried to actively silence what was happening in the gloomy cloud of pointing fingers loudly at others.

In 1943 the first corpses were discovered and exhumed, and the Soviets pointed to the Germans as the perpetrators. This could be substantiated as German weapons had been used. However, the details were not yet known. Officially, Poland and the Soviets were not yet in a declared state of war, and the relationships between their armies were undefined. More interested in silencing the events were the British and the US governments during the war, afraid of upsetting the Soviets as allied forces. The Germans were well-known to have established a brutal and horrible regime in Poland with countless atrocities; more than four million Polish citizens were killed or died during the German occupation.

After the war, pointing to the Soviets as perpetrators of the Katyn Massacre counted as pro-German. During the war, Polish accusations against the Soviets were used as an excuse to end diplomatic connections with the government in exile in London. The perpetrators established a "counter-trauma narrative" (Bartmanski & Eyerman, 2013, p. 239).

They managed to set in motion a knowingly false attribution of perpetrators and concealed the facts over an extended time. They conclude: "… we claim that a distinctive characteristic of traumatic narratives is an asymmetrical relation between perpetrator and victim and that this, in part, is what makes cultural trauma" (ibid.).

The physically embodied trauma is overshadowed by cultural trauma. It silenced over a long time what could be known, what was remembered, and what was only passed on in whispers. After Stalin died in 1953, a thaw initiated by Khrushchev's speech at the 20th Party Congress of the Communist Party made some cautious talking about Katyn possible and shifted responsibilities from the Germans to the Soviets. The whispers became audible beyond the circle of close family members, creating a dissonance between state guidelines and social life in affected families. As late as July 1988, the existence of confidential documents about the Katyn crime was denied. The whisper swelled into a scream.

> This cry for recognition was a signifier of a secretly lived trauma expressing a deeply suppressed "we," and the response of the authorities clearly showed that they too cared very much about the incident (…) the authorities sought to erase the remembrance of Katyn. (Bartmanski & Eyerman, 2013, p. 253)

The visit of Pope John Paul II in 1978 had started a discourse about the Katyn Massacre without permission from the authorities. Then, during the thaw after 1989, a scream arose in Poland. The Soviet authorities became insecure about what was permitted to say and what was not. Katyn—this became something so mighty, it was recognised as an undeniable fact. Other extermination sites like Mednoe and Kharkiv were included in public discourse. Katyn became visible and talkable. However, it remained without punishment for the perpetrators. The fight for the right to speak became complemented by hearing silencing.

"Nestbeschmutzer"

Another form of silencing closely relates to conformism: make no noise, smile, engage only in small talk, and behave as usual. These were the efforts of all who wanted to have what in the German vernacular of the

1950s was called a "Persilschein": a certificate that one has not been in a leading position, that one was a "little follower", and that, therefore, one was "not guilty of anything".[2]

The silencing in the Nazi period started with the "Hitler salute", a diabolic invention which unleashed an influence permeating everyday life in every corner. By forcing people to perform it, the *triviality* of a greeting was placed under the control of reciprocal observation. And more, the *personal* greeting and its variants became risky. In personal greetings, the Other is addressed. Gazes, body posture, and distances display a full range of expressions related to how two people define and experience their relationship. This observation does not exclude more formal greetings. But the enforced salutation does neither refer to nor recognise the other person, as both unify and devote their greeting to the dictator not present. And more, everyone could document loyalty to the leader and at the same time control the loyalty of the other. Mutual loyalty control and being under control became a trap that was not easy to escape.

This practice did not arise unexpectedly. It was the political programme of psychic expropriation. "There are no free spaces where the individual belongs to himself, the time of personal happiness is over, we will feel a community happiness." You do not belong to yourself. With these words, the president of the National Socialist Women's League, Gertrud Scholtz-Klink, had formulated the goal of destroying the emotional foundations of personal relationships (quoted in Allert & Chase, 2008). During the war, the propaganda minister, Goebbels called out: "They will never become free again"—from NS influences.

Let us follow some steps of how the re-appropriation of oneself was attempted.

Maria Ritter (2014, p. 187) is a psychoanalyst who emigrated to the US. She remembers that in the 1950s when she was in the third grade, she "… saw a flickering black and white film of the liberation of Auschwitz as part of a school-required denazification program." So attempts were present as early as the 1950s.

Charlotte Beradt (1966) gathered dreams people had in the Nazi period. She titled her book *The Third Reich of Dreaming*. These dreams

---

[2] "Persil" was the name of a detergent that promised the whitest possible laundry, and the expression "Persilschein" parodied the mad desire to "whitewash" perpetrators.

document that people felt observed and monitored, even in their most private areas; brushing their teeth, on the toilet, in bed—the manifest dreams showed them what was being politically planned and executed.

The strong influence of Alexander Mitscherlich is also to be mentioned. As a young doctor of medicine, Mitscherlich had the opportunity to observe the Nuremberg trials of the doctors of the Nazi party who had performed medical experiments on humans. Later, as a psychoanalyst and founder of the Sigmund Freud Institute in Frankfurt in 1960, he and his wife wrote books which strongly influenced public discourse in the sense of "coming to terms with Germany's past". The authors used psychoanalytic knowledge to make it understandable to a broader audience why Germans had these difficulties in mourning and being ashamed. It is not an exaggeration to say that these psychoanalytic texts strongly influenced the need to come to terms with the past as a new self-understanding of the new German republic. As a result, historians and philosophers (e.g. Voegelin, 1964) loosened their tongues and, in turn, contributed to the reconstruction and consolidation of a democratic conception of state and society that the Nazis had radically destroyed.

It is disconcerting to observe today that these early attempts at "working through" are too easily forgotten. The often-heard thesis that facing the horror has become possible "only now"—that is, in the third generation—is undoubtedly wrong. Many initiatives came from democratic parties, influential persons who returned from exile, trade unionists, and individual teachers. There were brave lawyers like Attorney General Fritz Bauer, who, in the early 1960s, brought to trial several of the concentration camp guards, SS men, and other guards from Auschwitz. The trials are in the cultural memory laid down as the "Auschwitz trials".

One outstanding achievement was in the 1990s the "Wehrmachtsausstellung" (exhibition of photographs made in the 1940s by German soldiers fighting in the Soviet Union), organised by the Hamburg Institute for Social Research initiated by Jan Philip Reemtsma. Many photographs of German soldiers in their military activities were documented—and many grandchildren discovered that what they saw was their grandfather involved in activities like hanging people. This exhibition generated tremendous reverberations in the German media. Sons and daughters of Nazi perpetrators, like Reinhard Heydrich, broke away from their families and wrote down impressive experiences of their lives with parents of that kind (Heydrich & Heydrich, 2012).

Nevertheless, one might wonder whether these efforts initiated by the cultural elite and governments reached the everyday lives of ordinary German families with their different and often troubling histories during the horrifying historical period.

Walking around the centre of Berlin, one cannot but notice large and striking memorials to the victims of National Socialist cruelties: murdered Jews, Roma and Sinti, homosexuals, and psychiatric patients. Although this was an admirable effort of German and Berlin authorities, one question remains: did the last of the memorials mentioned above open in 2014, sixty-nine years after the end of the Second World War, because it was easier to open discussions in and write for small circles than to build something that will be a reminder all the time, every day, and every night, to millions of passers-by?

It is well known that in the first period after the war, silencing was practised by labelling those who "desilenced" the Shoah and genocides as "Nestbeschmutzer". This word indicates that someone criticises his in-group—family, town, class, community (literally: pollutes his own nest). It was used as an accusation even in the German Parliament. It did not stifle the voices of Adorno and Jaspers, two well-known philosophers, but what was its influence on the millions of families around the country?

Two academic books have recently approached the latter of these questions, both with the help of psychoanalysis, on the other side of the ocean, and more than seventy years after the war.

The first one was written by Roger Frie, whom we proudly count among the contributors to this volume. The title of that book—*Not in My Family. German Memory and Responsibility after the Holocaust* (2017) cannot be more suggestive. Canadian of German descent, born in 1965, Frie suddenly found himself forced to resolve difficult questions. Is it the case that we readily recognise responsibility and guilt in our nations, tribes, and even neighbours but stop at the front door and deny seeing it in our most intimate groups? Frie precisely discovered this to be the case, and not in a large-sample research study but when by accident he saw a photograph of his beloved grandfather, a man whom he remembers as loving and with admiration of his generosity and infectious humour, in a paramilitary uniform, unmistakably connected with the Nazis. Doubts and guilt transform into research and writing, and the reader is presented with such frank and profound insights:

> On a bookshelf, I saw dusty copies of what I much later came to recognise as publications of the Nazi Party. They lay in a book-case full of classic works of German literature. Even after all this time, writing these words is highly discomforting. It is a history I do not wish to recognise, let alone share. I wrote, deleted, and rewrote the sentence about the Nazi publications several times before leaving it in place. Shameful feelings. The words on the page are now an unmistakable reference point connecting my personal history with the history of my family and Nazi Germany—intertwined, inseparable. (p. 195)

The second book is by Angelika Bammer, who was born in Germany immediately after the war's end, lived in Canada while her father worked in the German embassy, and moved to the US as a student. Titled *Born After. Reckoning with the German Past* (2019), the book contains a complex narrative built on personal memories, family photos, correspondence, and diaries, as well as the use of scholarly sources about this historical period and quoting Paul Celan, Theodor W. Adorno, and Walter Benjamin, three highly prominent names in working through the twelve years of National Socialism in Germany. Bammer is equally candid and deals unflinchingly with her father's mobilisation during operation Barbarossa and both her grandmothers' membership in the Nazi organisation for women. She also offers many gems of insight similar to this one:

> It was easy for me to blame my parents for their silence. For my post-war German generation, blame was the stance of choice. But I seldom asked them questions in ways that allowed for listening. I was too angry or afraid to grant what might have been their truth. Judging was easy. Empathy was harder. The understanding was almost out of reach.
>
> While my mother was alive, I was unwilling to hear what she might have told me. My eagerness to blame her silenced us both, and by the time I was ready to listen it was too late. (p. 231)

In Germany, Beate Niemann published the painfully revealing *My Good Father: My Living with His Past. A Biography of a Perpetrator* (2005). After decades of denial, she collected evidence of the thousands of deaths her father organised and commanded as chief of the Gestapo in Belgrade, Vienna, and Hungary. Once the book was published, she was criticised and even attacked by German right-wing political parties, and she decided to publish *I Do Not Permit Forgetting. NS-Past in Families' and Collective Memory* (2017). Similarly, journalist and author Alexandra Senfft wrote about her grandfather's responsibility (as ambassador in Slovakia) for the death of 70,000 Jews and his execution on the gallows in 1947. Her *Silence Hurts* was published in 2007. Over the years, so many people from around Germany approached her with their own stories that she published the 589-page long *The Long Shadow of the Perpetrators: Descendants Confront Their Nazi Family History* (2016).

From Mafia to FBI

To break the silence of at least one witness is essential for prosecutors. It has been achieved in the case of Luigi Bonaventura, a former mafia criminal. In an interview (Klaubert & Bonaventura, 2021), he formulates the reason for his turnaround: "The others shoot at you, at your family. So, you defend yourself by shooting at them, at their friends. Dead on one side, dead on the other. And in the end, you realise that there is only another 'you' lying on the ground." Another "you". "You" equals "me". This is the decisive discovery. Or denial. You shoot, and, in the end, you shoot yourself. Perpetrators destroy this basic rule of encountering social life (Goffman, 1961).

The cases that cause the most significant problems for the American FBI are when they find a body for which there seems to be no personal environment, no personal relationships, and no witnesses. No one can say anything, and no one can testify about anything. This, in turn, gives the investigators illegitimate opportunities. Another danger arises. That is why a bad word about J. Edgar Hoover, chief of the FBI, has been handed down from President Truman: "Once out of office, Truman confided to a friend that J. Edgar Hoover should be trusted 'as much as you would trust a rattlesnake with the silencer on its rattle'" (Hamm & Spaaij, 2017, p. 238). A silencer on the rattle is an impressive metaphor for what we are dealing with here. The rattlesnake warns by rattling its tail. Philomela could have heard the rattlesnake speaking, "… the captive has no chance". In Ovid's days, the same logic was used in not prosecuting committed crimes. Hearing silencing turns to a second field of interest: hearing silenced rattlesnakes.

However, if we lived in a world where we could not distinguish silenced rattlesnakes from police officers doing their job, we would be forced to conclude that we live in the most totalitarian states ever. It is not only that violence = love, that police officers = rattlesnakes, and judges = enemies. It is that your language turns into something you cannot trust. You learn "double talk", as George Orwell named it in *1984*, or a "double language". You change your memories to "screen confessions", where you do not refer to your memory but "to how it is constructed in language":

> Not the concrete facts are omitted from these confessions (therefore they are completely reliable in terms of their factual value), but their deep meaning. Distortion or error, here, does not inhere in the concrete details but in the syntax which interferes in different ways with the original utterance, removing its deep meaning even if all of its components are accurate and correct. (Amir & HaCohen, 2020, p. 298)

What you get to hear is on the surface. People confess things they never have committed. They turn into rattlesnakes without having a poisonous tooth in their mouth.

Silencing perpetrators

As Macbeth testifies, the first danger against silence comes from the perpetrator himself. The rapist of Philomela is tormented by his conscience, and Macbeth loses his mind and can only go on murdering because he follows the logic of "silencing the witnesses". Of course, neither of them acts without being tormented by conscience, but quite the opposite is true. From these artistic representations and historical experiences, mafia-like organisations conclude that one must oblige the perpetrator himself to remain silent. It is better not to kill him, as he might still be needed, but to oblige him to participate. Only when he has killed someone must he be aware that the others know that he has become committed. And his commitment can be believed. As a witness, he would not only incriminate others but always himself as well. The most important task, then, becomes to silence yourself.

Wilhelm Hauff—Abner the Jew who has seen nothing (1827)

Wilhelm Hauff's narrative work is concerned with a satirical circumvention of censorship in Germany in the early nineteenth century, at the time of the Restoration period ordered by Metternich in 1815. The novella *Abner* exposes oppositional liberal-democratic tendencies and philosemitic visions. Consequently, Hauff's novella is to be read in the context of the oppositional German Vormärz (1815–1848). Hauff's novella *Abner* was published in his second *Almanac* of novellas in 1827. The setting of the story is Morocco. After a hard day's work, the Jewish physician and merchant Abner is calmly going for a walk in a small wood of palms and dates. He wants to relax after a busy day. Suddenly the emperor's henchmen on horseback approach him aggressively. They ask Abner whether he has seen the noble horse and the empress's runaway noble bitch. Abner describes the two animals to them accurately. He tells the henchmen what the animals look like and shows them the direction in which they escaped from the disciplinary imperial house, an indirect reference to the situation of Jews in early nineteenth-century Germany. That is the reason why Hauff places the narrative in Morocco. Hauff's narrative programme is called covert narration because it challenges the reader to uncover allusions on the level of meaning (Ramm 2022). Because Abner is a Jew, the guards do not believe him. They ask Abner whether he really saw the noble animals. Abner ironically and with self-confidence replies that he has *not* seen them, but the guards should search in the direction he indicated.

> "A small quail dog," Abner continued, "recently whelped young, long coat, feather tail, limps on the right foreleg." "She is as she lives and breathes" cried the chorus of blacks, "it is Aline; The Empress went into convulsions as soon as she was missed; Aline where art thou? what shall become of us if we return to

the harem without thee? Speak quickly, where did you see her run off?" "I have seen no dog at all, for I do not even know that my empress, whom God bless, possesses a quail's dog." Then the people of the stables and the harem were enraged at Abner's impudence, as they called it, in joking about imperial property. (Hauff, 1970, p. 141)

The horse riders find the animals and lead them and Abner to the emperor. The emperor is pleased about the return of his noble animals because his politics revolve around them—Hauff's satire of dictatorship in the early nineteenth century. At the same time, the emperor is annoyed with Abner, who tells him that he has *not* seen the animals. By now, the readers are as irritated as the henchmen and the emperor. The readers fall into the trap of this novella. Abner self-confidently explains to the emperor that he has deduced their direction from the web of tracks the animals have left on the ground and the bushes where they have fled. As a reward, Abner receives one hundred strokes on the soles of his feet, some money, and a pardon for his exposure of a personal privilege of the emperor, which the emperor cultivates instead of engaging in responsible politics. In the second part of the novella, this pattern is varied. If one deciphers Hauff's covert narrative, which none of the censors in Hauff's time succeeded in doing, then it becomes clear that Abner shrewdly makes visible what is kept politically invisible. This applies to the politics of the emperor, as well as to Abner, to the narrator Wilhelm Hauff, and to the reader, who were able to decipher Hauff's story. Hauff satirically exposes the foolishness of dominating powers who promoted the unnatural stereotyping and social exclusion of Jews at the beginning of the nineteenth century and who had critical works censured. Hauff mockingly highlights the humanity of Abner, the physician and merchant, against the emperor and his henchmen.

Charles Dickens: *Oliver Twist* (1837–1839)

In Charles Dickens's second novel, *Oliver Twist*, the focus shifts in the first third of the plot from the main character Oliver to Nancy, a prostitute who wants to protect Oliver from being murdered by the pimp Sykes.

Sykes is connected to Fagin's gang of thieves. Nancy overhears a conspiratorial meeting and reveals it to Mr Brownlow, who also wants to protect Oliver. This conversation is overheard by a boy in the band of thieves, who passes it on to Sykes via Fagin. Sykes brutally murders Nancy. He silences her so that she will not betray the band of thieves, Fagin, and himself, all criminals. At dawn, Sykes rushes to Nancy. He is furious:

> The housebreaker freed one arm and grasped his pistol. The certainty of immediate detection if he fired, flashed across his mind, even in the midst of his fury, he beat it twice with all the force he could summon, upon the upturned face that almost touched his own. She staggered and fell, nearly blinded with the blood that rained down from a deep gash in her forehead, but raising herself with difficulty on her knees, drew from her bosom a white handkerchief (…) and holding it up in her folded hands as high towards Heaven as her feeble strength would let her, breathed one prayer of mercy to her Maker. It was a ghastly figure to look upon. The murderer staggering backwards to the wall, and shutting out the sight with his hand, seized a heavy club and struck her down. (Dickens, 1841, Book III, chap. 9, pp. 396–397)

The murder has a terrible effect on Sykes. He flees and sees visions and is convinced Nancy's corpse is following him. Her eyes follow him everywhere:

> And here he remained in such terror as none, but he can know, trembling in every limb, and the cold sweat starting from every pore, when suddenly there rose upon the night wind the noise of distant shouting, and the roar of voices mingled in alarm and wonder. (Dickens, 1841, Book III, chap. 10, pp. 402–403)

Sykes's extreme mental state, expressed in his body language, reveals his murder of Nancy to the readers, and it reveals to them that Sykes does not know himself anymore, a scene similar to Shakespeare's mad King Lear. However, contrary to the deliberate murder of Nancy, Sykes bears witness to his deed in his body language. He lost self-control; he has lost himself.

The murder is discovered. Sykes now flees across the rooftops of London and strangles himself unintentionally. The murderer silences himself. Charles Dickens took Shakespeare's plays as models. These can be understood as narrative transformations of Shakespeare's tragedy *Othello* (1603/1604) into Victorian criminal milieus as explored and published by Dickens in the early 1820s as a young and still unemployed court reporter.

The author himself is the imaginative witness who knows and narrates Nancy's murder. Literary critic Terry Eagleton understands the world of Dickens's novels thus: "The point of a Dickens novel may lie in its formal narrative, but most of its life is to be found lurking in its margins and subtexts" (Eagleton, 2008, p. 152). That is, Dickens's subtexts reveal what is concealed in Victorian society. Dickens speaks, as a witness, about exploitation, violence, crime, and sexuality. His novels are paradoxically structured by seemingly disconnected coincidences but have secret affinities. His novels reverse the patterns of concealment. His novels depict: "… a great deal *about* the streets, raising caricature, grotesquerie and broad-brush-portraiture to a new kind of artistic perceptions" (Eagleton, 2008, p. 162). By appealing to the readers' implicit knowledge, Dickens transforms readers into witnesses, too. Dickens tells and plays a paradox in front of his audiences: what is concealed cannot be silenced. One truth about his protagonists is a core theme of modern literature and culture: they never arrive at themselves. Their possibilities of developing an autonomous personality are thwarted by violence and silencing. Polanski's film version of *Oliver Twist* also focuses on the view of the persecuted and the victims.

Chimamanda Ngozi Adichie: *Purple Hibiscus* (2003)

Nigeria's new literature deals with British colonialism and its consequences. Adichie's novel is in dialogue with Chinua Achebe's novel *Things Fall Apart* (1958). Achebe's novel explores the social, cultural, and religious life of an Igbo village with patriarchal structures and crises before and after the confrontation with colonialism in rural Nigeria. Adichie's novel confronts in an urban milieu a fanatical Christian religiosity converted from Igbo culture (through the protagonist Eugene) with the vibrancy of modernised Igbo culture (through Eugene's antagonist Ifeoma). The plot spans three years. Adichie's novel is set in the educated black African middle class in the Nigerian city of

Enugu and in the Nigerian university town of Nsukka, which is bio-graphically the place of Adichie's family. While Achebe's novel *Things Fall Apart* deals with the disruption of pre-modern African cultural conditions by colonising patterns in relation to Igbo culture, Adichie's novel *Purple Hibiscus* interprets the impact of this cultural transforma-tion on a modernised Igbo culture torn apart, as a failure (Eugene) and as a living togetherness (Ifeoma). That is the geopolitical background of this novel. The title *Purple Hibiscus* can be understood as a symbol of love, freedom, and resistance.

Kambili is Eugene's fifteen-year-old daughter and first-person nar-rator of the novel. Eugene is the patriarchal head of the family, of the Christian Igbo. Eugene's family lives in Enugu. Eugene's liberal-minded sister Ifeoma lives in Nsukka. She is Eugene's antagonist. Eugene is a strict Catholic who has internalised the norms of the colonial rulers. He uses authoritarian and sadistic methods to force his wife, Kambili, and her brother Jaja to submit to the rituals of the Catholic Church and thus to him. He beats them up like mad. In the process, his wife, who endures everything, suffers at least two miscarriages. Eugene also scalds the feet of his children. The first-person narrator is stunned and, like her mother and brother, retreats into silence, a narrative outcry that pervades the novel:

> I cleared my throat, willed the words to come. I knew them, thought them. But they would not come. The sweat was warm and wet under my arms. (Adichie, 2003, p. 64)

An indirect witness to the abuses and degradations is Ifeoma. She knows her brother, sees through him and his sadistic outbursts, and reads what has happened from the children's and their mother's body language. Their body language witnesses Eugene's cruelties and makes them public. Ifeoma is a university lecturer and single mother of three children. She courageously confronts Eugene's sadistic rituals and grad-ually helps Kambili and Jaja become independent personalities who learn to take responsibility for themselves. Before this, there is a horrific scene in which Eugene beats Kambili to the point of needing hospi-tal treatment, because she and Jaja are looking at a painting depicting their deceased Igbo grandfather. It is Eugene's father whom he denies because he has not converted to the Catholic faith. Kambili is already lying on the ground to protect the painting Eugene tore up:

> "Get up! Get away from that painting!" I lay there, did nothing. "Get up!" Papa said again. I still did not move. He started to kick me. The metal buckles on his slippers stung like bites from giant mosquitoes. He talked nonstop, out of control, in a mix of Igbo and English, like soft meat and thorny bones. Godlessness. Heathen worship. Hellfire. The kicking increased in tempo, and I thought of Amanka's music [Ifeoma's daughter], her culturally conscious music that sometimes started off with a calm saxophone and then whirled into lusty singing. I curled around myself tighter, around the pieces of painting; they were soft, feathery. They still had the metallic smell of Amanka's paint palette. The stinging was raw now, even more like bites, because the metal landed on open skin on my side, my back, my legs. Kicking. Kicking. Kicking. Perhaps it was a belt now because the metal buckle seemed too heavy. Because I could hear a swoosh in the air. A low voice [Kambili's mother] said, "Please, *biko*, please." More stings. More slaps. I closed my eyes and slipped away into quiet. When I opened my eyes, I knew at once that I was not in my bed. (Adichie 2003, p. 255)

As the fifteen-year-old Kambili narrates the horrific events, Adichie's novel expresses a paradox that exacerbates the concealment of family tyranny in the 1990s as a reflection of a (Nigerian) society where a corrupt military dictatorship ruled until 1999. Moreover, the paradox of vulnerability is instantiated through the female child protagonist of Adichie's novel. In this sense, "… her presumed innocence makes her a powerful and harmless vessel of domestic and societal vicissitudes" (Coker, 2017, p. 101).

Kambili represents a challenge to the status quo. On the same level against the status quo is Beatrice, Kambili's and Jaja's mother. After losing at least two babies because Eugene brutally beats her up and being unable to protect herself and her children from Eugene, she eventually ends the cycle of violence by gradually poisoning Eugene. Jaja takes the blame for his mother's deed and goes to prison. His likely liberation offers Beatrice some hope at the end of the novel. Jaja takes responsibility for his father's death and himself.

In the subtext of Adichie's novel lurks an energy of protest that expresses itself in its language. The aesthetic atmosphere of Adichie's novel illuminates that the use of the Igbo language within the narrative shows appreciation for this element of African heritage. This affirmation is vital in the novel's postcolonial context. An African language is proudly appreciated in the literature and defended with some reservations against the societal and historical status quo. That is empowering. Adichie tells of deliberately induced atrocities that silence the victims of her novel and colonial history, which in turn is kept quiet by the perpetrators. Adichie writes against degradation. In terms of colonial history, the world watched the atrocities out of greed for profit and power. Adichie's novel is a globally relevant political testimony of systems of injustice that conceal their murderous intentions and deeds. Her novel makes these concealments visible.

In the literary texts discussed, the body language of the perpetrators or the victims reveals the concealment of inequitable or criminal and murderous acts. The critical question is the following: do dictators with high utilitarian intelligence have a low threshold sense of responsibility? Or do they *decide* to silence others to be able to commit their acts?

Invasions

In October 2021, during the COVID-19 pandemic, the first news leaked that Russia had assembled large masses of troops at the border with Ukraine. A lot of diplomatic, political, military, and secret services activity followed, about which most citizens were informed very roughly. The outlet for the news was a permanent denial from the Russian side that attacks against Ukraine were intended. In January and more in February 2022, Russian speakers used the term "Western hysteria". The war began on February 24, 2022.

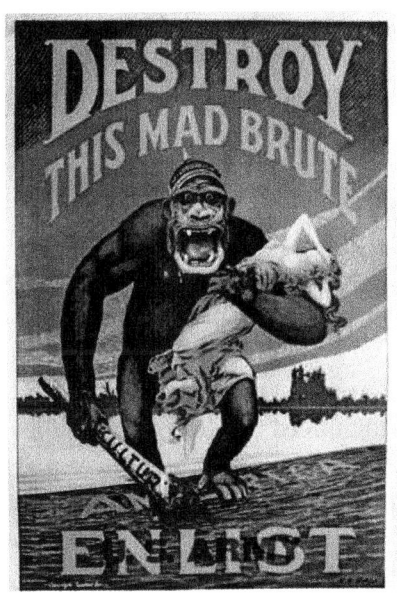

One message stood out. Two weeks before the invasion, Putin, in a political statement (Busse, 2022), named Ukraine "My beauty" who will have "to bow down", which meant "to submit" or "to comply"—a clear allusion to sexual male phantasies—to take the woman *a tergo*. We easily identify the fraudulent embellishment (rape disguised as love), the "hunting", a metaphor, and the promise of a solemn act (the purification of Ukraine from "Nazis"). This quote about "beauty" disappeared in television and radio news, and in newspapers, it was silenced.

Nevertheless, there is a multitude of forerunners in which territorial conquests are presented as conquests of a woman: rapes. The German soldier of the First World War was depicted as a club-wielding King Kong, carrying conquered Belgium in the form of a ravished woman in his arms. American propaganda depicted the German beast on a poster by Harry Ryle Hopps in 1917 aimed at motivating mobilisation for the US entry into the war.

The difference is that Putin ascribes the rape to his side in the fight. It is a call to his people, an invitation to rape, which could have taken Aaron's call in Shakespeare's *Titus Andronicus* as a model. Aaron invites his men:

AARON:
> My lords, a solemn hunting is in hand;
> There will the lovely Roman ladies' troop.
> The forest walks are wide and spacious,
> And many unfrequented plots there are,
> Fitted by kind for rape and villainy.
> (Shakespeare, *Titus Andronicus*, 1:608–612, The New Oxford Edition)

This is Aaron's *call* for a gang rape. Here are the single elements which constitute the perceptible gestalt of the call: "hunting" is promised, added by a fraudulent embellishment, "solemn". Ultimately, the cat comes out of the bag: "rape and villainy". Lovely Roman ladies are announced for the hunt, and the places are promised as wide and spacious. Again, this a fraudulent embellishment: lovely ladies implicitly are turned into whores. The next element: Aaron describes the sites as "unfrequented"—implicitly, he promises no witnesses. Shakespeare lets

Aaron present all elements as "opportunity": no witnesses, lovely ladies, vast space, and a metaphorical contradiction—solemn hunting. Thus, it becomes possible to describe rape publicly as a solemn act. In the same moment and move, what can be heard is silenced.

Putin uses a metaphor of love, turning his intentions into being well meant and peaceful. But the second part, "the beauty" has to "comply", announces *and* hides the violence set in action as self-ascription is historically new and that betrays a guilty conscience. Putin describes his war party in metaphors formerly used *against* enemies. This might have contributed to his metaphorical call for rape being widely silenced in public attention. Putin's call was heard but did not lead to the conclusion that it was a call to his men.

This is not the case with Russia only. There are too many countries and governments one could point to. We want to contribute to open ears for the incredible, unbearable number of violent acts happening worldwide at every moment. They can be heard and seen; they are not "unconscious". Those who suffer are silenced. And vice versa, those who are silenced suffer from missing an ear that can hear.

Conclusion

Of all the forms of silencing, the most dramatic may be the silencing of abuse victims. Though the silencing performed by religious or educational institutions is no doubt more comprehensive, most of the time, it "goes under the radar" and can easily be taken for granted. But when another person, including children or a group, becomes a victim of torture, images and impressions are powerful and long-lasting. Especially if silenced, victims will probably bear pain inside themselves throughout their lives and this will result in developmental disorders.

Witnesses remain or are forced to be silent all too often because they believe that protects them. After all, it is too challenging to keep observing, because of shame, intimidation, and denial. We choose silence for ourselves and those we live with and love, whereas the audacity to speak up is rarely cultivated. Finally, not only victims, but even perpetrators can be and often are silenced to be made obedient and collaborative.

It turns out that silencing follows violence almost inevitably and that we are all at least sometimes silenced—a grim image which we might be tempted to avoid. Yet no matter how little we are focused on it, it will never loosen its grip on our lives.

References

Achebe, C. (1958). *Things Fall Apart*. New York: Penguin, 2017.

Adichie, C. N. (2003). *Purple Hibiscus*. Stuttgart, Germany: Reclam, 2019.

Allert, T., & Chase, J. (2008). *The Hitler Salute: On The Meaning of a Gesture*. New York: Metropolitan Books/Henry Holt and Company.

Amir, D., & HaCohen, N. (2020). Screen confessions: The test case of "breaking the silence". *International Journal of Applied Psychoanalytic Studies, 17*(4): 296–312. https://doi.org/10.1002/aps.1649

Bammer, A. (2019). *Born After: Reckoning with the German Past*. New York: Bloomsbury.

Bartmanski, D., & Eyerman, R. (2013). The worst was the silence: The unfinished drama of the Katyn massacre. In: R. Eyerman, J. C. Alexander, & E. Butler Breese (Eds.), *Narrating Trauma. On the Impact of Collective Suffering* (pp. 237–267). Boulder, CO: Paradigm.

Beradt, C. (1966). *Das Dritte Reich des Traumes (The Third Reich of Dreaming)*. Munich, Germany: Nymphenburger.

Busse, N. (2022, February 11). Putin's Säbelrasseln. *Frankfurter Allgemeine Zeitung*.

Coker, O. (2017). The paradox of vulnerability: the child voice in *Purple Hibiscus*. In: E. N. Emenyonu (Ed.), *A Companion to Chimamanda Ngozi Adichi* (pp. 101–113). Rochester, NY: Boydell & Brewer.

Danieli, Y. (1984). Psychotherapists' participation in the conspiracy of silence about the Holocaust. *Psychoanalytic Psychology, 1*(1): 23–42. https://doi.org/10.1037/0736-9735.1.1.23

Dickens, C. (1841). *Oliver Twist*. London: Penguin, 2003.

Dimitrijević, A. (2020). Silence and silencing of the traumatised. In: A. Dimitrijević & M. B. Buchholz (Eds.), *Silence and Silencing in Psychoanalysis. Cultural, Clinical, and Research Perspectives* (pp. 198–215). London: Routledge.

Dimitrijević, A., & Buchholz, M. B. (Eds.) (2020). *Silence and Silencing in Psychoanalysis. Cultural, Clinical, and Research Perspectives*. London: Routledge.

Eagleton, T. (2008). *The English Novel: An Introduction*. Oxford: Blackwell.

Figes, O. (2008). *The Whisperers: Private Life in Stalin's Russia*. London: Penguin.

Frie, R. (2017). *Not in My Family: German Memory and Responsibility After the Holocaust*. New York: Oxford University Press.

Goffman, E. (1961). *Encounters: Two Studies in the Sociology of Interaction*. London: Penguin University Books.

Grand, S. (2013). *The Reproduction of Evil: A Clinical and Cultural Perspective*. Relational perspectives book series. Hoboken, NJ: Taylor and Francis.

Hamm, M. S., & Spaaij, R. (2017). *The Age of Lone Wolf Terrorism: Studies in Transgression*. New York: Columbia University Press.

Hauff, W. (Ed.) (1970). *Sämtliche Werke, Band II, Märchen, Novellen*. Stuttgart, Germany: Deutscher Bücherbund.

Heydrich, L., & Heydrich, H. (Eds.) (2012). *Mein Leben mit Reinhard: Die persönliche Biographie* (2nd edition) (*My Life with Reinhard: The Personal Biography*). Gilching, Germany: Druffel & Vowinckel.

Jack, D. C., & Ali, A. (Eds.) (2010). *Silencing the Self Across Cultures: Depression and Gender in the Social World*. New York: Oxford University Press. https://doi.org/10.1093/acprof:oso/9780195398090.001.0001

Klaubert, D., & Bonaventura, L. (2021, November 1). "Man wächst als Kindersoldat auf". Der Kronzeuge Luigi Bonaventura über seine Kindheit in einer 'ndrangheta-Familie, den eigenen Aufstieg zum Boss und die Konequenzen seines Bruchs mit der kalabrischen Mafia. *Frankfurter Allgemeine Zeitung*.

Lyotard, J. F. (1988). *The Differend: Phrases in Dispute*. G. Van Den Abbeele (Trans.). Manchester, UK: Manchester University Press.

McAffee, M. (2016). Rephaim, Whisperers, and the Dead in Isaiah 26:13–19: A Ugaritic Parallel. *Journal of Biblical Literature*, *135*(1): 77–94. https://doi.org/10.15699/jbl.1351.2016.3022

Mucci, C. (2013). *Beyond Individual and Collective Trauma: Intergenerational Transmission, Psychoanalytic Treatment and the Dynamics of Forgiveness*. London: Karnac.

Niemann, B. (2005). *Mein guter Vater: mein Leben mit seiner Vergangenheit: eine Täter-Biographie* (*My Good Father: My Living with His Past. A Biography of a Perpetrator*). Berlin: Hentrich & Hentrich.

Niemann, B. (2017). *Ich lasse das Vergessen nicht zu. NS-Vergangenheit im familiären und kollektiven Gedächtnis* (*I Do Not Permit Forgetting. NS-Past in Families' and Collective Memory*). Berlin: Lichtig.

Ovid. *Metamorphoses*. A. D. Melville (Trans.). The World's Classics. Oxford: Oxford University Press, 1986.

Pröll, F. (2022, January 4). Kämpfen ohne Hände (Fighting without hands). *Frankfurter Allgemeine Zeitung.*

Ramm, Hans-Christoph. (2022). *Wilhelm Hauff—Spiele des Bösen. Die Märchenalmanache, Mitteilungen aus den Memoiren des Satan, Das Bild des Kaisers.* Darmstadt: Wissenschaftliche Buchgesellschaft.

Ritter, M. (2014). Silence as the voice of trauma. *American Journal of Psychoanalysis, 74*(2): 176–194.

Senfft, A. (2007). *Schweigen tut weh: Eine deutsche Familiengeschichte* (*Silence Hurts: A German Family History*). Hamburg, Germany: Claassen.

Senfft, A. (2016). *Der lange Schatten der Täter: Nachkommen stellen sich ihrer NS-Familiengeschichte* (*The Long Shadow of the Perpetrators: Descendants Confront Their Nazi Family History*). Munich, Germany: Piper ebooks.

Voegelin, E. (Ed.) (1964). *Hitler und die Deutschen* (*Hitler and the Germans*). Munich, Germany: Wilhelm Fink.

CHAPTER 2

"But break, my heart, for I must hold my tongue": examples of self-silencing in classical and contemporary literature

Aleksandar Dimitrijević and Michael B. Buchholz

Introduction

If we think about silencing, we mostly turn to examples of forceful influence on individuals or whole groups by other individuals or groups. Although these may be the most obvious examples, and they are indeed quite frequent, in this chapter we want to turn to self-silencing, a phenomenon of no lesser consequences. Persons in various roles may decide not to share their experiences with anyone due to shame, fear, pride, or the lack of language necessary for description (for more details see Dimitrijević, 2020). We will use three masterful literary descriptions, which, although coming from different eras and genres, offer profound and textured explorations of this process.

Hamlet

An incredible number of human problems or ideas can be related to *Hamlet* as their prototype or even their source, and it seems that the phenomenon of silencing is one of them. Just as countless other interpretations of the play and its main character(s) have claimed that it was all about melancholy (e.g. Jenkins, 1982, pp. 106–108;

see also Dimitrijević, 2015), overthinking (e.g. the interpretation offered in Goethe's novel *Wilhelm Meister's Apprenticeship and Travels*, later supported by Coleridge and many others), Protestantism (e.g. Greenblatt, 2001; 2005, pp. 288–322), the Oedipus complex (e.g. Steiner, 1994),[1] and many other concepts, it can be shown that it is (also) about silencing.

Hamlet explicitly deals with speech, hearing, and silence. The word "silencing" is present in this most abundant treasure trove of the English language. We learn that there are "golden words" (V.2, 129)[2] as well as "pestilent speeches" (IV.5, 91), that it is possible to "speak daggers" (III.2, 387), and if you "lend thy serious hearing" (I.5, 5) Hamlet has "words to speak in thy ear [that] will make thee dumb" (IV.6, 22–23).

From the very first scene, this concern is everywhere. Characters have problems communicating with one another—"ears, that are so fortified against our story" (I.1, 34–35)—and suddenly have to communicate with no less than a ghost: "If thou hast any sound or use of voice, speak to me" (I.1, 131–132). But when the Ghost refuses to address the guards, they decide to alert Hamlet believing that it is the ghost of his father: "This spirit, dumb to us, will speak to him" (I.1, 176). Indeed, the motif of silencing culminates with the Ghost's description of purgatory:

> But that I am forbid
> to tell the secrets of my prison house,
> I could a tale unfold whose lightest word
> Would harrow up thy soul, freeze thy young blood,
> Make thy two eyes like stars start from their spheres,
> Thy knotted and combined locks to part,

---

[1] A bibliography of psychoanalytic texts about Shakespeare for more than fifteen years contained 461 items (Willbern, 1980), and the number has constantly been rising. In two methodical book-length overviews, Philip Armstrong (2001) introduced the expression "psychoanalytic Shakespeare", and Carolyn Brown (2015) wrote about "Shakespearean psychoanalytic criticism".

[2] All quotations from *Hamlet* are taken from the second Arden series edition (ed. Harold Jenkins).

And each particular hair to stand on end
Like quills upon the fretful porpentine.
But this eternal blazon must not be
To ears of flesh and blood.

(I.5, 13–22)

Ghost here deploys a strategy we can discover in many (though certainly not all) instances of what is termed intergenerational transmission of trauma. First, he declares that he is himself silenced ("forbid"), then he uses the strongest possible figures of speech to destroy the peace of mind and inflame the imagination of the person he is allegedly protecting, to end by repeating that he is not allowed to say anything. It is inevitable that all the horrors he has listed will remain imprinted in his son's mind tenfold.

But even with his mind on fire, Hamlet does not forget that he must treat everything as a secret. Before he had any word about or from the Ghost, he had proclaimed the motif of the whole play—"But break, my heart, for I must hold my tongue" (I.2, 159)—and asked Horatio to "let it be tenable in your silence still; And whatsoever else shall hap tonight, give it an understanding but no tongue" (I.2, 248–250). And what he learns from the Ghost he will not share with anyone but his tablets.[3]

Where does this concern come from? Hamlet must have suspected early on and gathered more and more evidence that Denmark was full of people who called themselves "lawful espials" (III.1, 32). Polonius is most devoted to this and advises his son to "give thy thoughts no tongue (I.3, 59) ... give every man thy ear, but few thy voice; take each man's censure, but reserve thy judgement" (68–69). Claudius then asks Rosencrantz and Guildenstern to seduce Hamlet into revealing his mind, hoping that Hamlet is "easier to be played on than a pipe" (III.2, 361). To Claudius's great disappointment and concern, Hamlet keeps his secret, and the spies can only report that he "will by no means speak. Nor do we find him forward to be sounded, but with a crafty madness

---

[3] Although "tongue" is used here more metonymically, we know that Shakespeare was aware of the practice of silencing via actually cutting or plucking people's tongues (see our chapter on silencing victims in this volume).

keeps aloof when we would bring him on to some confession of his true state" (III.1, 6–10).

As if this does not suffice, different characters are silencing one another throughout the play. Hamlet makes Horatio and the guards swear they will "never make known what you have seen tonight" (I.5, 149). While Claudius wants Hamlet silenced utterly and plots his death, to stop Hamlet's accusation Gertrude exclaims "no more" four times: "O speak to me no more. These words like daggers enter in my ears" (III.4, 94–95). Even poor Ophelia is followed at the King's command and the effects of her condition on the general public are closely monitored (IV.5).

Hamlet has over the last two centuries attracted much attention because of the postponement of revenge and consequential self-exploration and self-criticism. Immediately after the meeting with the actors, Hamlet speaks about the pressure of his self-imposed silencing. Instead of revenge, he "must like a whore unpack my heart with words" (II.2, 581) and not revealing the truth to anyone, he says in the soliloquy, "O what a rogue and peasant slave am I!" It is important to note that Hamlet does not talk to himself for a hypertrophy of self-reflection,[4] that will later be praised by the Romantics. Soliloquies, considered by some to be Shakespeare's greatest theatrical invention (see Greenblatt, 2005, pp. 298–311), for Hamlet are a mere necessity: he simply cannot and dare not trust anyone and talks to himself because in Elsinore even walls have ears. He is silenced by the oppression of his uncle's rule and Polonius's espionage. He speaks his mind only after he can say "Now I am alone" (II.2, 543).[5]

This combination of silencing and self-silencing is so unbearable that it becomes uncertain how long Hamlet can survive it. Doing what

---

[4] Harold Bloom calls Hamlet "the prince of interiority" (1998). This reading was strongly emphasised already in Bradley (1904) who influenced all subsequent Shakespeare scholars.

[5] This is emphasised very strongly in the 1964 film version directed by Grigori Kozintzev. Renowned for the fine acting by Smoktunovsky and the music score by Shostakovich, the film portrays Hamlet walking through masses of people and saying the soliloquies only in his mind. Soviet artists obviously knew a thing or two about risks involved in telling the truth as did everyone in the state of "whisperers" (Figes, 2008).

his father did to him, he will use non-verbal signals, make another person deeply upset and silenced, and get temporary relief by overwhelming another. This is what we learn from Ophelia about Hamlet's state of mind and behaviour presumably just after he heard the Ghost's story.

> My lord, as I was sewing in my closet,
> Lord Hamlet, with his doublet all unbrac'd;
> No hat upon his head; his stockings foul'd,
> Ungarter'd, and down-gyved to his ankle;
> Pale as his shirt; his knees knocking each other;
> And with a look so piteous in purport
> As if he had been loosed out of hell
> To speak of horrors, he comes before me. (II.1, 77–83)

> He took me by the wrist and held me hard.
> Then goes he to the length of all his arm;
> And with his other hand thus o'er his brow,
> He falls to such perusal of my face.
> As he would draw it. Long stay'd he so.
> At last, a little shaking of mine arm,
> And thrice his head thus waving up and down,
> He rais'd a sigh so piteous and profound
> As it did seem to shatter all his bulk
> And end his being. That done, he lets me go,
> And with his head over his shoulder turn'd,
> He seem'd to find his way without his eyes,
> For out o' doors he went without their help,
> And to the last bended their light on me. (II.1, 88–100)

Because of this and Hamlet's later explicit abandonment of her in the "get thee to the nunnery" scene, Ophelia will lose the capacity to speak intelligibly and eventually possibly kill herself by drowning. Her final statements and singing bear the resemblance of speaking but she is actually silenced in a more profound way than Hamlet as she is devoid of meaning—"Her speech is nothing" (IV.5, 7). Silence is not hers originally, it was given to her by Hamlet, who in turn had received it from his father's ghost.

There is a serious hint that total silencing is impossible: "for murder, though it have no tongue, will speak with most miraculous organ" (II.2, 589–590). But such optimism may be alien to a tragedy. Hamlet seems to find his new voice in the graveyard of all places. First, he mourns the loss of Yorick, whose "skull had a tongue in it, and it could sing once" (V.1, 74). Then he jumps out of Ophelia's grave to proclaim, "This is I, Hamlet the Dane!" (250–251). This will not last long, and sensing that he is dying, Hamlet asks Horatio to tell his story: "Report me and my cause aright to the unsatisfied (V.2, 343–344) … things standing thus alone, shall I leave behind me (350) … tell my story (354) … tell him, with the occurrents more and less which have solicited—the rest is silence" (362–363).

But even Horatio does not know the whole story, as he did not hear crucially important details Hamlet said only in soliloquies (see Dimitrijević, 2022). Claudius and Gertrude are both already dead, as is Polonius, and Fortinbras does not seem to be interested in asking questions. The true story is, thus, destined to remain untold, silenced, from the viewpoint of the play's characters, although readers and spectators can be overwhelmed by it.

Stalingrad

An impressive novel published in 1952, *Stalingrad* tells us a lot about self-silencing in a different context. The author, Vassily Grossman, was a Soviet war correspondent from the beginning of the German invasion in June 1941, who wrote poignantly about the suffering of the Soviet people. He was close to the front lines and wrote a great many reports, often speaking with fighting soldiers in whose dugouts close to the front he stayed. His novel itself has a publication history that fits into our theme. It was published, retracted, revised again, put into translations that were then not permitted by the political censors, and was published in English in 2019 and in German in 2021. What Grossman describes is the course of the war. But above all, he impressively describes what people experience under such horrific circumstances, their suffering, their heroism, their struggle and—their silence and being silenced. On both the Soviet and German sides.

The first example is about a German soldier. We quote an editorial note. Schmidt was on sentry duty and worries about falling asleep, which might betray him as disloyal, filled his thoughts. In an afterword, the editors sum up the various versions of Grossman's writing:

> Grossman's response exemplifies his ability to make creative use of editorial interference. In the third version and 1952, Schmidt thinks, "Or he might mutter something incorrect in a dream. His neighbour would hear him, wake some of the others and say, 'Here, listen to what this red Schmidt has to say about our Führer.'" Here Grossman simply transliterates the word "Führer." In 1954 this sentence ends with the words "listen to what this red Schmidt has to say." And in the 1956 edition it ends with the words "listen to what this red Schmidt has to say about our Leader." This time, however, the word for "leader" is "vozhd"— the usual Soviet way of referring to Stalin. This whole passage, therefore, can be read as a statement not only about life in Nazi Germany but also life in Soviet Russia. (Grossman, 2019, p. 1009)

It is easy to understand that Schmidt is a German soldier who, while falling asleep, is described as thinking about his thoughts—how to get them under control? What Grossman makes of this is a literary description of a true dimension: Schmidt fears his thoughts—why? Because he might be discovered to equalise Stalin and Hitler as the same type of oppressors, dictators.

In another scenario, we follow a Russian scientist at a Moscow institute, Victor Shtrum, who remembers how a befriended scientist, Maximov, made a scientific tour through those countries that were occupied by Germany before the attack on Russia. The biochemist Maximov, a representative of a large academic faculty, reports at the Moscow institute on a trip through Czechoslovakia. This country had been conquered by the Nazis, but Russia had not yet been invaded. Maximov says that people were so afraid to speak, the scientists there asked Maximov not to ask them any questions. Below is what Shtrum says about the former friend:

> He's the head of an important faculty, but he behaves like some petty criminal, afraid the police might collar him at any moment. "Don't ask me anything at all," he said. "It's not only my colleagues I'm afraid of. I'm afraid of my own voice. I'm afraid of my own thoughts." (Grossman, 2019, p. 223)

In the period between the non-aggression pact (August 23, 1939) and the German invasion of the Soviet Union (June 22, 1941), Stalin suppressed all criticism of Nazi Germany and Hitler. By recalling this episode so candidly from his former friend, Maximov put himself in danger. Those who try to free themselves from the web of self-entanglement easily run the risk of becoming entangled in it.

In the second volume of this novel, Shtrum is in danger of finding his voice again. He made significant discoveries in physics and is elected to win the Stalin prize. But his findings contradicted the doctrine of Marxism-Leninism. The staff of the institute arrange that the prize is withdrawn. Others, even close friends, distance themselves from him, the caretaker no longer greets him, and acquaintances cross the street to avoid meeting him.

He goes through a very difficult period of isolation. His wife also isolates herself from him. But he wants to hold on to his findings. He has a dark suspicion that something could come out of it that will be significant for the arms industry. One evening, when he is at home, he receives an unexpected phone call—from Stalin himself! The conversation lasts barely three minutes: Stalin wants to wish him success in his work.

The wind has changed. Suddenly, the old contacts are re-established, people greet him, and he is celebrated. Everything seems normal. Shtrum realises how much he is in danger. He wants to rejoice, to bask in the protection of the powerful. But he knows well enough: "One word from Stalin could destroy thousands and thousands of people" (p. 923).

He must remind himself, admonishingly, not to lose his mind. He must keep his own voice silent.

The Human Stain by Philip Roth

An excellent contemporary example of self-silencing is the central theme of Philip Roth's The Human Stain.[6] This novel, published for the first time in the year 2000, contains many layers: it is at the same time about politics at large and university politics, about racial and sexual

---

[6] Psychoanalysts have also shown a lot of interest in Roth's novels (just as he has frequently written about psychoanalysis). For a contemporary review of The Human Stain see Buchholz, 2001, and for an overview, Scheurer, 2015.

relationships, sexual abuse and war trauma, parents and children, age gaps, and much more. Most of all, though, it is about Coleman Brutus Silk, a professor of classics, once a powerful and dynamic college dean, relentless in pursuit of academic excellence. Silk resigns after a ridiculous charge of racism is taken seriously by his colleagues, and then his wife of more than forty years, the mother of his four children, suddenly dies. Furious because he believes she was murdered by those who conspired against him and those who chose to be comfortably silent, he asks Roth's (probable) alias to write his story to save it from silence.

Silk tried to write the book himself for no less than two years but now finds the draft useless. Its tentative title is "Spooks", which is how it all began. When a couple of students were constantly absent, he asked the class, "Are they real or are they spooks?" and was accused that he did not mean "ghosts" but "niggers".[7] The question is, however, why an experienced language professor was unsuccessful in writing his own story.

Our narrator, Zuckerman, will discover only near the very end of the sequence of events, Silk's story, or at least its official version, which was never complete. Considered by everyone to be Jewish and buried after a religious ceremony in a synagogue, Silk was an African American of fair complexion, "lily-white", as his elder brother once tried to offend him, and he built his entire inner and social life around hiding this. He silenced one side of his identity, and a defining one in American society at that. Silk never shared the secret with his wife or children, or with a single one of his friends and colleagues.

This "self-fashioning" began in the years immediately after the Second World War, and almost incidentally. While still a high school kid in New Jersey, Silk turned out to be not only a valedictorian student but also a promising boxer nicknamed Silky Silk. His coach wanted to help him get a "boxing scholarship" for a prestigious university, where Silk would not have been accepted because of the then rampant racism:

> "If nothing comes up," Doc said, "you don't bring it up. You're neither one thing nor the other. You're Silky Silk. That's enough. That's the deal." (...)

---

[7] This episode was based on a real-life experience of a friend of Roth's (2012) and seems even more significant today when all aspects of academia are politicised.

"He won't know?" Coleman asked.

"How? How will he know? How the hell is he going to know? Here is the top kid from East Orange High, and he is with Doc Chizner. You know what he's going to think if he thinks anything?"

"What?"

"You look like you look, you're with me, and so he's going to think that you're one of Doc's boys. He's going to think that you're Jewish."

This planted seeds in Silk's mind. He acutely felt, from his own and his father's experiences, that he would always be stigmatised, always belong to a large group in the eyes of other people, and always be a part of either "we" or "they". But his father fell one day during his shift as a waiter in a dining car and died much before his time, and the son, still in his formative years, sensed his loss opened the door for a unique opportunity:

Only with his father in the grave did Coleman at last bother to hear them—and when he did, instantaneously to aggrandize them. This had been purposed by the mighty gods! Silky's freedom. The raw I. (...) Overnight the raw I was part of a we with all of the we's overbearing solidity, and he didn't want anything to do with it or with the next oppressive we that came along either. (...) He was Coleman, the greatest of the great pioneers of the I. (...) No. No. He saw the fate awaiting him, and he wasn't having it. Grasped it intuitively and recoiled spontaneously. You can't let the big they impose its bigotry on you any more than you can let the little they become a we and impose its ethics on you. Not the tyranny of the we and its we-talk and everything that the we wants to pile on your head. Never for him the tyranny of the we that is dying to suck you in, the coercive, inclusive, historical, inescapable moral we with its insidious E Pluribus Unum.[8] (...)

---

[8] This Latin phrase means "to make one out of many" and is the unofficial motto of the USA.

Instead the raw I with all its agility. Self-discovery—that was the punch to the labonz. Singularity. The passionate struggle for singularity. The singular animal. The sliding relationship with everything. Not static but sliding. Self-knowledge but concealed. What is as powerful as that? "Beware the ides of March."[9] Bullshit—beware nothing.

The first significant experiment occurred when Coleman enlisted for service in the army, checking the box "White". The next one was only partly successful, when after the war, in New York City, he dated all sorts of girls until he brought one of Scandinavian descent and a Minnesotan upbringing to meet his mother and sister. The now popular phrase, "He happens to be black" was indeed applicable to Coleman, yet with other family members, there was no doubt about their origin. The girl found this too much and, in tears, left him.

Cherishing the development of his "raw I" higher than anything, he thus concluded that no future girlfriend could ever be allowed to meet his family, nor will the wife, children, grandchildren, friends … He had to sever his ties with them and his past completely. And doing that, he also severed his ties with himself. He "managed to force himself to ignore his feelings, whether of fear, uncertainty, even friendship—to have the feelings but have them separately from himself", and discovered that "there is the drive to master things, and the thing that is mastered is oneself". He became a self-proclaimed "self-freedom fighter" with "an actable self, big enough to house his ambition and formidable enough to take on the world".

Outwardly, Coleman planned and executed everything perfectly well, to the level that, afraid one of his kids might look "openly black", he married a Jewish girl.

---

[9] Julius Caesar was killed on the Ides of March, a holiday that took place on March 15. The very phrase "Beware the Ides of March" comes from Shakespeare. In the eponymous play, Caesar is warned by a prophet and then reminded of it by his wife, Calpurnia. However, he decides not to pay attention, goes to the Senate, and is killed, on Largo Argentino, by some of his closest friends and collaborators. It is certainly significant that Silk was named after one of Caesar's murderers and the main character of Shakespeare's play.

> He wondered if this entire decision, the most monumental of his life, wasn't based on the least serious thing imaginable: Iris's hair, that sinuous thicket of hair that was far more Negroid than Coleman's (...) crazy fear that all that he had ever wanted from Iris Gittelman was the explanation her appearance could provide for the texture of their children's hair (...) he had the definite impression that he had just chosen a wife for the stupidest reason in the world and that he was the emptiest of men.

He proceeds with symbolically killing his mother. In a conversation that is one of the highlights of this superbly written novel, the widowed woman, to whom he was always the apple of her eye, now learns that she will have to disappear from his life and never meet him or his (future) children:

> "You're never going to let them see me," she said. "You're never going to let them know who I am. 'Mom,' you'll tell me, 'Ma, you come to the railroad station in New York, and you sit on the bench in the waiting room, and at eleven twenty-five A.M., I'll walk by with my kids in their Sunday best.' That'll be my birthday present five years from now. 'Sit there, Mom, say nothing, and I'll just walk them slowly by.' And you know very well that I will be there. The railroad station. The zoo. Central Park. Wherever you say, of course, I'll do it. You tell me the only way I can ever touch my grandchildren is for you to hire me to come over as Mrs Brown to babysit and put them to bed, I'll do it. Tell me to come over as Mrs Brown to clean your house, I'll do that. Sure, I'll do what you tell me. I have no choice."

He intentionally "let her continue to employ her words to absorb into her being the brutality of the most brutal thing he had ever done. He was murdering her." And the intention was clear:

> ... only through this test can he be the man he has chosen to be, unalterably separated from what he was handed at birth, free to struggle at being free like any human being would wish to be free. (...) It's so awful that all you can do is live with it. (...) Once you've done a thing like this, you have done so

much violence it can never be undone—which is what Coleman wants. (...) If in the service of honing himself, he is out to do the hardest thing imaginable, this is it, short of stabbing her. This takes him right to the heart of the matter.

And he perseveres with the plan to the very end of his life, replying to all enquiries that he was the only child of early deceased parents and "that he was Jewish, Silk being an Ellis Island[10] attenuation of Silberzweig, imposed on his father by a charitable custom official".

But one has to wonder why all this was necessary, and what the purpose of this whole identity change was. And therein lies the psychological core of Coleman Silk as a character (and the reason for this brief review):

> How did such a man as Coleman come to exist? What is it that he was? Was the idea he had for himself of lesser validity or of greater validity than someone else's idea of what he was supposed to be? Can such things even be known?

If it were ambition only, lusting for success with the list of women worthy of Don Giovanni, or if it were well-known greed and envy, all histories would have been resolved quickly. Silk wants all of this and, at the same time, much more, or better put, he wants the top prize that human existence can come up with:

> The confidence right in his bones to be his particular I. Free on a scale unimaginable to his father. As free as his father had been unfree. Free now not only of his father but of all that his father had ever had to endure. (...) Free to go ahead and be stupendous. Free to enact the boundless, self-defining drama of the pronouns we, they, and I.

This level of freedom comes at the price of burning all bridges, not only towards his mother and siblings but also his past, memories, and identity. We learn a lot about dean Silk, but not that he was a creative scholar

---

[10] A small island off Manhattan, where ships from the Atlantic entered the US and used to bring many immigrants.

who developed his intellectual passions. We learn equally much about Coleman as a private person, but not that he loved his wife passionately, that he played with his kids selflessly, or that he took care of his mother furtively. The reason for this probably lies in the fact that

> he became not just an unknown but an incohesive person. In what proportion, to what degree, had his secret determined his daily life and permeated his everyday thinking? Did it alter over the years from being a hot secret to being a cool secret to being a forgotten secret of no importance, something having to do with a dare he'd taken, a wager made to himself way back when? (...) By the time I met him, was the secret merely the tincture barely tinting the colouration of the man's total being or was the totality of his being nothing but a tincture in the shoreless sea of a lifelong secret? Did he ever relax his vigilance, or was it like being a fugitive forever?

The dark tones of the second half of the novel suggest the later interpretation. The only detail Zuckerman seems to forget is that Silk was also a fugitive from his own self.

Roth offers us three possible metaphors of Silk as a person. First, most obviously, the bird raised in a cage, about whom the phrase "the human stain" will first be used. When allowed to fly out, it is attacked by other birds because its voicing is developed as the imitation of children's imitations of bird voices. Forced to grow in captivity, it could not belatedly become free. Metaphorically speaking, it failed where Coleman hoped to succeed. Second, his Athena college is reformed thanks to his ambition and iron will, but it will betray him by the end. And finally, the frozen lake where Les Farley, the traumatised Vietnam veteran whose driving led to Silk's death, fishes through tiny holes,[11] and although an excellent metaphor for the US as a society (portrayed throughout the novel with merciless honesty and criticism), may also be

---

[11] "There it was, if not the whole story, the whole picture. Only rarely, at the end of our century, does life offer up a vision as pure and peaceful as this one: a solitary man on a bucket, fishing through eighteen inches of ice in a lake that's constantly turning over its water atop an arcadian mountain in America."

seen as a psychological report about Coleman Silk, whose authenticity froze and could be evoked only at rare and strange moments.[12]

If this interpretation of the novel's end makes sense, it confirms that Silk's mother was right all along, when she said, "You think like a prisoner. You do, Coleman Brutus. You're white as snow and you think like a slave."

Because Silk strived towards absolute social freedom at the cost of fundamental personal slavery, and an opportunity to have his professional stance heard far and wide at the cost of having his intimate voice stifled by his own decision, he oversaw that the core of human freedom was in the articulation of all voices one contains, and, like Oedipus, ended at the place from which he had most valiantly tried to escape.

Conclusion

We have seen that the process of self-silencing can be initiated by intense external pressures—emotions like fear, shame, embarrassment, or wish to protect someone—as well as by inner insecurities, lack of self-confidence, and loneliness, or by one's secret decisions related to ambition.

We reviewed just three examples of self-silencing from the literature. Their divergence—one coming from Early Modern England, the other from the post-Second World War Soviet Union, and the final from the US at the turn of the millennia—seems to suggest that the phenomenon was well-known to artists. Add to this list Chief from Ken Kessey's *One Flew Over the Cuckoo's Nest* or a host of Kafka's short stories in which the protagonist turns into a mute/subhuman character, and you will be tempted to think that self-silencing is rather universal.

The question we are left with is why psychology and psychoanalysis have not recognised and described this process much earlier.

---

[12] His late relationship with Faunia Farley, thirty-seven years his junior, passionate and stormy though it undoubtedly was, Roth all too often compares to the relationship Aschenbach has with the thirteen-year-old Tadzio of Thomas Mann's *Death in Venice*. Hence, one can conclude that Roth indicates that the affair reflects dissolution rather than love.

References

Armstrong, P. (2001). *Shakespeare in Psychoanalysis.* London: Routledge.

Bloom, H. (1998). *Shakespeare: The Invention of the Human.* New York: Riverhead.

Bradley, A. C. (1904). *Shakespearean Tragedy.* London: Macmillan.

Brown, C. (2015). *Shakespeare and Psychoanalytic Theory.* London: Bloomsbury.

Buchholz, M. B. (2001). Review of Roth, Philip: *The Human Stain. Psyche,* 55(12): 1332–1335.

Dimitrijević, A. (2015). Being mad in early modern England. *Frontiers in Psychology,* 6: 1740.

Dimitrijević, A. (2020). Silence and silencing of the traumatised. In: A. Dimitrijević & M. B. Buchholz (Eds.), *Silence and Silencing in Psychoanalysis: Cultural, Clinical and Research Perspectives* (pp. 198–215). London: Routledge.

Dimitrijević, A. (2022). Historical roots of solitude and private self (with continual reference to Shakespeare). In: A. Dimitrijević & M. B. Buchholz (Eds.), *From the Abyss of Loneliness to the Bliss of Solitude* (pp. 57–68). Bicester, UK: Phoenix.

Figes, O. (2008). *The Whisperers: Private Life in Stalin's Russia.* London: Penguin.

Greenblatt, S. (2001). *Hamlet in Purgatory.* Princeton, NJ: Princeton University Press.

Greenblatt, S. (2005). *Will in the World: How Shakespeare Became Shakespeare.* New York: W. W. Norton.

Grossman, V. (2019). *Stalingrad.* Robert Chandler and Elizabeth Chandler (Trans.). New York: New York Review of Books.

Jenkins, H. (1982). Introduction. In: W. Shakespeare, *Hamlet* (pp. 1–159). London: Arden.

Roth, P. (2012, September 6). An open letter to Wikipedia. *The New Yorker.*

Scheurer, M. (2015). "What it adds up to, honey, is homo ludens!": Play, psychoanalysis, and Roth's poetics. *Philip Roth Studies,* 11(1): 35–52.

Steiner, R. (1994). In Vienna veritas …? *International Journal of Psychoanalysis,* 75: 511–583.

Willbern, D. (1980). A bibliography of psychoanalytic and psychological writings on Shakespeare, 1964–1978. In: M. M. Schwartz & C. Kahn (Eds.), *Representing Shakespeare: New Psychoanalytic Essays* (pp. 264–286). Baltimore, MD: Johns Hopkins University Press.

CHAPTER 3

Traumatic disclosures and failures of listening

Stephen Frosh

Silencing

This chapter is not about silence, which can be healing and comforting as well as disturbing or eerie. It is, rather, concerned with acts of *silencing*, which always implies a situation in which something that needs to be heard is refused, or someone who wishes to speak is denied that opportunity. Silencing is an act of *suppression*; silencing of dissent is only the most explicit way in which this occurs (tanks in the square, water cannon on the street, government functionaries in the courts), but there are other ways too, such as deliberately turning away from someone who is speaking, or loudly interrupting them, or prematurely claiming to understand what one doesn't understand at all. Is silencing through suppression ever appropriate? Debates regarding what to do about hate speech, racial abuse, and outrageous political lying and incitements to violence—"injurious speech" (Butler, 1997)—are complex and range from allowing it to be expressed by refuting it, to criminalising it. This is an increasingly difficult issue in a political context in which right wing populism, and the lies attendant upon it, are prevalent, linked in brutal ways with authoritarianism and intolerance. Should all speech be encouraged so that no important things are left unsaid, or are there limits to what is tolerable and, if so, how do we decide what they are? Making decisions about this might not seem so difficult if we are discussing genocidal advocacy or homophobic hate, for example, but what about hurtful speech that stops short of the outright lies, racist conspiracy theories, and belligerent provocations which run rife over the public sphere? I will leave it to legal and ethical theorists to deal with this, only to note that any simple idea that all silencing is wrong might need to be considered carefully and critically.

Silencing can involve inventing a myth that there is only silence when in fact there has been a lot of unheard, unlistened-to noise, which elsewhere I have named as "murmuring" (Frosh, 2019), but this might in fact be a direct communication that is simply denied by the recipient ("nobody said anything"). For example, the claim that Holocaust victims were silent for twenty years or so after the end of the Second World War is not true to what happened, which is that many of them spoke out through testimonies and extensive writings in Polish and Yiddish at the end of the 1940s and early 1950s. The problem was not that there was silence, but that there was little response to this speaking and, as a result of this, the survivors' voices dried up (Cesarani & Levene, 2002). Even one of the most celebrated and influential of Holocaust memoires, Primo Levi's *If This Is a Man*, was not "heard" when first published by a small Italian publisher in 1947, when it sold only 1500 copies; it did not gain traction until the end of the 1950s. That is to say, the text was there, but few people read it; the difficulty of communicating trauma was not that it could not be articulated, but that this articulation was avoided or denied.

One might say similar things about the issue concerning disclosures of child sexual abuse and generally, the responses to child abuse. There had been very little registration of the frequency of sexual abuse until it burst on the therapeutic and political scene in the late 1970s and 1980s (at least in the UK, my setting), yet it rapidly became clear that this was not because no one had reported it but because the voices of children and women were systematically stifled by the lack of response to their calls. This social deafness was aided by a misreading of psychoanalytical ideas but, more generally, was produced by a misogynistic culture adept at assuming that women and children (and women treated as children) had nothing to say of value. The flood of disclosures that subsequently arrived revealed not only the prevalence of child sexual abuse but the many attempts that children and women had made to be heard, only to be met with silence or active rejection. As Sándor Ferenczi (1949) pointed out a very long time ago (actually in 1932, demonstrating that the "secret" of child sexual abuse has been in plain sight for the best part of a century), sexual abuse of children is much more common than was believed to be the case. After discussing how the abused child might react with anxiety, guilt, and identification with the abuser, he comments on the role of the "second adult", the one who receives a full or partial disclosure, usually the parent or sometimes the psychoanalyst.

> Usually, the relation to a second adult—in the case quoted above, the mother—is not intimate enough for the child to find help there, timid attempts towards this end are refused by her as non-sensical. The misused child changes into a mechanical, obedient automaton or becomes defiant, but is unable to account for the reasons of this defiance. His sexual life remains undeveloped or assumes perverted forms. (Ferenczi, 1949, p. 228)

This might have too many echoes of the assumptions of its day (the neglectful mother, the language of "perversion") but the broader point remains important: the "second adult", the one who does not hear the screams or whispers of distress, contributes significantly to the disturbance that sexual violence causes. The timid attempts of children to transmit information about what has happened to them will require adults to increase the volume on their receivers; instead, however, they commonly refuse to hear anything and treat the message as nonsensical. That is indeed a way to silence someone effectively.

Sometimes, psychoanalytically, silencing involves *repression*, denial, foreclosure, or some other unconscious technique that ensures that a troubling voice is left unheard, or a disturbing idea is nipped in the bud. For Jean Laplanche, famously, this is as true of psychoanalysis as it is of humanity in general; indeed, it is a psychoanalytic truism that we back away from the disturbing things we almost know, including knowledge itself. Laplanche (1999) calls this psychoanalysis's tendency towards "going astray" from its own most radical insights. Using Freud's idea that he was the Copernicus of psychology, revealing how each of us is not the centre of our universe, Laplanche comments:

> If Freud is his own Copernicus, he is also his own Ptolemy. The revolution in astronomy lasted nearly two millennia, with some intuitions of the truth almost from the start, but also with an initial going-astray. In psychoanalysis everything, essentially, is produced by a single man—*simultaneously: the discovery*, affirmed at a very early stage, and which is conjointly (and for me indissociably) that of the unconscious and that of seduction—*and the going-astray*, the wrong path taken each time there was a return to the theory of self-centring, or even self-begetting. (Laplanche, 1999, p. 60)

Laplanche's idea of the relation between the unconscious and "seduction" might be important here, but for the moment the more relevant point is his reference to the "wrong path" taken by Freud and by psychoanalysis generally. For Laplanche, this particularly signifies loss of the radical awareness of the causal role the "other" plays in the formation of the human subject, how difficult it is to resist the temptation to "return to the theory of self-centring", to make everything relate to the subject rather than to the other. More generally, it states what seems to be a universal truth, both discovered and enacted by psychoanalysis, that whenever we get close to exposing ourselves to difficult knowledge, the kind of knowledge that disturbs us—for example, knowledge of trauma, whether our own or someone else's—there is a huge temptation to back away. This kind of silencing may well be unconscious and may even *produce* the unconscious, in the sense of creating a class of things (ideas, memories, desires) that we know and don't know at the same time (the "unknown knowns", to use the fourth, unmentioned, pole of Rumsfeld's famous schema). The thing that speaks inside us, that *speaks to us* as psychoanalysis might conceive of it, is by its very nature (the nature of the unconscious) the thing we least want to hear. This refers both to our own inner realities, if I can use that formulation, and to what comes at us from "outside". It means, therefore that we might abhor in the other what disturbs us in ourselves.

Faced with the traumatised other, we might respond by a mode of traumatic identification, in which we act as if we ourselves have been traumatised. This can function as a mode of silencing because it means that we do not make ourselves available as a separate entity to be "used" by the other in the sense that Winnicott (1969) describes such use as a resilient "object" available to bring something *different* to the encounter rather than simply mirroring the other's distress and in that way augmenting it. This augmentation can happen, for instance, by making the "other" responsible for the trauma inflicted on our self by simply witnessing *their* trauma. Responding to a trauma testimony by becoming traumatised ourselves ("Yes, yes, I know how awful it is, it is so terrible. Similar things happened to me!") might seem like an empathic way to react, but it means that the listener has vacated the crucial position of witness and become another victim, *claiming* the speaker's distress rather than responding to it. As such they become "useless" as a separate "object" who might offer help. Alternatively, we might respond by turning away, self-protectively or out of guilt at feeling implicated in the trauma. This is an even more explicit rejection of the speech of the traumatised subject even if its reality is acknowledged ("I can't listen to you, it is too much for me") and even more so if it is doubted ("It can't have been like that, you are misremembering or misrepresenting what happened," and so on—though the witness's capacity to remain capable of independent *thinking* is also critically important). The term "implicated" used just above is not an accident either. Understanding that the position from which we witness another's suffering is not neutral is itself both an important ethical stance and an uncomfortable realisation that can lead to defensive silencing. Indeed, while acknowledging that we are always "implicated" in the other's suffering might be crucial to developing a full response to it (Rothberg, 2019), *partial*, unworked-through awareness of implication can make it harder to find a way to witness another's trauma testimony, contributing in a major way to the process of silencing. A sense of implication leading to guilt as well as the difficulty of dealing with the emotions generated by other people's suffering can produce resistance to listening. To be clear, this is not an argument against awareness of implication; on the contrary, it is a statement about what can happen when our unconscious awareness of how implicated we might be in the situation of another as victim (of racism, for instance), is not allowed into awareness to challenge us, but remains an unconscious source of discomfort and is defended against by the wish to not hear what the other might be trying to say.

Déjà vu

The voices we try to silence keep finding ways of speaking, but it is also the case that the silencing process goes on and on just as repetitively, unless something breaks it. Psychoanalysis is quite clear about this: repetition occurs until a troubling issue is worked through; without such working through we are haunted by ghosts that cannot be laid to rest. "In an analysis", writes Freud (1909b, p. 123), "a thing which has not been understood inevitably reappears; like an unlaid ghost, it cannot rest until the mystery has been solved and the spell broken." Such hauntings, as I have tried to describe elsewhere (Frosh, 2013), are indications of a disturbance in the structure of the social world. Often this concerns forms of violence (ghosts frequently result from violent deaths) which take on the form of trauma. Yet these repetitions and returns are not exact; the things that keep on repeating, that seem to have happened before, are always different when they return. The fluidity of memory is a central claim of psychoanalysis, after all, codified in its version of temporality as a to-ing and fro-ing between past and present ("Nachträglichkeit"): all important things repeat and return, but every time they do so they are also different—reworked, in a new context, with new meaning attached to them that in turn creates new pasts and new futures. This is also a basic point about trauma, the concept perhaps most widely indexed in discussions of silence and silencing. Traumatic experiences keep coming back, as ghosts kept from resting in peace, because something has not been resolved, because some injustice continues to be unrecognised and unrequited (Gordon, 1997). Trauma itself is defined in this way, certainly within the psychoanalytically influenced literary "trauma culture" that has dominated much discussion of it in the social sciences over the past thirty years (Caruth, 1996). Here, the characteristics are usually given as some version of the following:

1. In contrast to conventional forms of narration or historiography which are linear, causal, and sequential, the temporality of trauma is characterised by repetition, circularity, or stagnation. Trauma leaves a person locked out of history in the sense that what returns is not experienced as *past* but instead as *immanent*, as overwhelmingly

present *in* the present. This results in a more general collapse of past and present, in opposition to the clear-cut separation of now from then held to be necessary for healthy functioning. As one psycho-analytic trope puts it (Loewald, 1960), the problem is of converting ghosts into ancestors, and this has not happened because the ghosts are unsatisfied and so cannot take their place in the proper chronology of grief and mourning. Their graves have not yet been filled in.

2. Because the experiences they describe are so difficult to grasp, over-whelming the subject's capacity to symbolise them, trauma testimonies are fragmented, cryptic, and muted—raising accusations of being incoherent, incomprehensible, and untrue. This relates to Dori Laub's (1992) somewhat overstated differentiation between narrative and historical truth (roughly translating to "subjective" and "objective" accounts of reality), but it also describes a certain kind of speech or writing, the performance of which attests to the presence of trauma. Indeed, the argument is circular: trauma leads to apparently incoherent testimony; incoherent (fragmentary, affect-full, or affect-less) testimony indicates the presence of trauma; speaking too coherently suggests something overworked and hence untrustworthy. We might note about this that the promotion of frag-mentation as the truth of all testimony, all narrative even, within much contemporary thought, sometimes as an aspect of decolo-niality but also of elite post-structuralist argumentation, is part of the evidence for the domination of a "trauma culture". There are no coherent narratives, or coherence in narrative is automatically sus-picious, given the realities of psychic and social complexity. Does this promote a "trauma consciousness" in itself? And does it, in an odd yet pervasive way, act against the interests of justice? In some rape and sexual abuse situations, legal presentations require a cer-tain kind of packaging for narrative sense to be made of trauma testimonies (Hlavka & Mulla, 2021). In court, this can confusingly demand that victims demonstrate *both* the performance of disor-ganisation *and* the integration of this disorganisation into a coher-ent story. Without the former, the narrative that is produced may be held to be overly well structured and therefore unlikely to repre-sent the reality of the trauma; but without the latter, the testimony may be regarded as unreliable and incomprehensible. The bind on

testimony and hence its likely silencing is therefore powerful; the straits through which a convincing narrative must be navigated are exceedingly constrained.

3. "As a relation to events, testimony seems to be composed of bits and pieces of a memory that has been overwhelmed by occurrences that have not settled into understanding or remembrance, acts that cannot be constructed as knowledge nor assimilated into full cognition, events in excess of our frames of reference." Shoshana Felman's (1992, p. 5) formulation, which this is, sums up the argument given above that trauma cannot be captured as memory, but swamps it, so testimony is bound to be fragmentary, and because of this easily denied or returned to its broken shape. The corollary of this is that trauma essentially cannot be spoken of, but only somehow communicated via an affect-laden incoherence which prompts a mirroring response in the interlocutor—a traumatic identification, in some cases. Felman writes (p. 16), "The testimony will thereby be understood, in other words, not as a mode of *statement of*, but rather as a mode of *access to*, that truth." To my mind, while this conveys something of the experience of receiving testimony, it is also a somewhat dangerous assertion, suggesting that trauma testimony can never be processed intellectually, but only received as a kind of affective bundle that strikes a chord in the listener. On the other hand, both Felman and Laub very importantly point to precisely this question of how a witness to testimony might respond to it in what, in lay language, one might call "emotional" ways, picking up the affective undercurrents of what might be halting speech. This can be very exhausting, and one might suggest, thinking of the formalities of court procedures as well as therapeutic encounters, that one response is to drain trauma talk of its affective harmonics so that listeners are spared its demands. This will then be another form of silencing: legal, didactic, and psychoanalytic speech might easily be a defence against the material itself, protecting witnesses to the testimony from having to undergo an experience of traumatic identification. Or, put more simply, this apparently "objective" speech is an intentionally distancing device serving the interests of justice less than those of psychic retreat.

4. But perhaps the main way of not listening to trauma is part of a very widespread problem with trauma discourse which assumes that the

difficulty of testimony is the lack or incoherence of speech, meaning that a trauma perseveres because it is not properly enunciated. In this model, trauma maintains its characteristic tendency to return and repeat precisely because it cannot be adequately symbolised by the sufferer and so is not properly "digested" or "worked through". As I have been arguing, the problem, however, may not be so much with the lack of speech on the part of the trauma victim or *its* incoherence; the problem seems much more intensely located in the lack of listening and the incoherence that so excruciatingly typifies the *response* to victim testimony. This is the main source of déjà vu: the ghost must keep battering on the door to gain access to a full hearing of its complaint, repeatedly reproducing both the trauma and the rejection unless something can be made to change. Too often, this is exactly what fails to occur.

Registering child abuse

My sense of something returning—my déjà vu, to keep to the occult frame of ghostliness—has a few different components, which came back to me in a flood when I participated in a round-table discussion of new research on sexual violence (SHaME, 2021). One of them is my own mini trauma from 1988, when a book I co-authored with Danya Glaser on *Child Sexual Abuse* was published in the UK, jointly by a commercial publisher and the British Association of Social Workers (Glaser & Frosh, 1988). In the theoretical section of this book, we examined the question of why it was (and is) primarily men who are abusers (at that time we thought this was almost universally the case, though this has to be tempered now) and argued that the answer lay in the sexual socialisation of men. My university put out a press release on this idea that patriarchal sexual socialisation links with abuse and a reporter from the British tabloid *Daily Mail* was immediately on my doorstep (literally, sitting there waiting for me to come home and helping me in with the shopping), with a front-page item the next day, headed "Doctors say all men are sex abusers." My fifteen minutes, or seven days, of fame followed, as the media (feeding off itself as it always does) took this up with enthusiasm, linking it to attacks on the family and the rise of a kind of radical feminism that had supposedly infiltrated welfare and psychiatric institutions, apparently posing a mortal threat to them. These were days when the culture wars that continue to rage over children, families, and women were at one of their regular high levels of intensity—then as now—and we were a kind of cannon fodder.

I raise this memory here because it came back when thinking about the question of how one might be silenced and how an important conceptual claim might be obscured or terrorised out of hearing. Here, the claim was about patriarchy and its concrete impact on the lives of men, women, and children; but elsewhere one might think the same things about "race" and the attempt to shut down critical race theory. Content might have changed, but the process of refusal to look at troubling truths, or at least ideas, continues. And there are many ways of doing this. Allow me another brief personal moment. Recently, I have been involved as a chair of governors with a local school. We had some issues of what is now called "safeguarding" relating to concerns over children involved in sexualised behaviour, and this resulted in referrals through the local Multi-Agency Safeguarding Hub or MASH as it is known. What struck me most was how little has changed in the last twenty years or so since I stopped doing child protection work in the English National Health Service. There is the same experience of confusion about what is "normal" sexual behaviour and what might be indicative of something pernicious happening; the same muddle about what should be reported to whom; the same leaking boundaries and uncertainty over lines of responsibility; the same mutual recriminations among professionals; and perhaps most of all the same defensive practices, in which urgent referral, case conferences, and erratic emergency action (almost always then dropped, leaving people in limbo) take the place of thoughtful, child-centred work. Child sexual abuse then and now has this capacity to promote moral panic and the terror of being found to have done something wrong—to have the blame slipped onto the professional—often leaving children who have been abused struggling, wondering who they might be able to trust.

My point is not that action should not be taken to protect children—quite the contrary—but that there are many ways to silence victims of abuse, including direct scaremongering and pillorying of those who try to think critically about issues that trouble a community or society at large, as well as creating procedures that mimic action but in reality achieve very little, what Sara Ahmed calls "non-performatives" (Ahmed, 2021). Behind this are various forms of defensiveness, especially denial. The most obvious methods with regard to sexual abuse involve discouraging and ignoring disclosures that come from children themselves. These disclosures often appear as hints and behavioural enactments that require interpretation and are therefore encased in doubt about what they could mean, creating uncertainty and anxiety and requiring careful and sometimes relatively slow assessment if they are to take the form of genuine witnessing. Disclosures also come sometimes from carers or observers of children, who themselves might be unclear about what they know and whose motives may occasionally be called into question. Such disclosures usually provoke intense activity in school or social care authorities, but this activity may raise hopes that something helpful will happen only to dissipate in muddle, lack of action, and very long-drawn-out yet inconclusive investigations. As Ferenczi (1949) pointed out, the end result is to discourage further disclosure and to build up a model of the world which is best described as "hypocrisy"—saying one thing ("We are here to help") and doing another.

The defensive structures of this lack of response include the kind of moral panic that denounces critical thought described in my *Daily Mail* experience above, which under the guise of "reporting" aims to mock and silence voices that dissent from normative assumptions about social practices—practices that preserve and reproduce traumatic experiences by refusing to examine their determinants. Official agencies also often institute silencing through non-performativity, by making it appear that something is being done when nothing significant is happening at all. These are at best strategies for ensuring that neither individuals nor society are troubled by the import of disclosure claims, until some crisis makes the defence unmanageable, and everything breaks down. At that stage, the system moves into gear to control and contain the crisis, someone is blamed, and silence returns to make everyone feel secure again. Perhaps the most famous example of this, at least in the UK, is the "Baby P" case of a child killed by his parents in 2007. This is documented by Sharon Shoesmith (2016), who at the time had been director of Children's Services for the relevant authority, and who was instantly dismissed by the then Secretary of State for Children and Families during a television interview. Shoesmith eventually took out a judicial review of her treatment and received compensation, but the damage was done—she was vilified, social workers across the country retreated into defensive practice in case the same happened to them, tabloid newspapers promoted visceral hatred of those trying to keep children safe, and children continued to be murdered every week. While this was not a sexual abuse case, many of the same processes apply: a sequence of missed opportunities for seeing or hearing a child's suffering; an eventual terrible event; and a social consensus to find someone to blame rather than examine the real sources of such suffering in social discrimination, inequality, poor funding of services, inadequate training and support for child protection workers, institutional confusion, and political demeaning of notions of "welfare". The silencing here is twofold: of the child's voice, for one, and of the murmur-turning-into-roar of social oppression, in which vulnerability is pilloried as weakness so that responsibility for it can be avoided, and, when this becomes unsustainable, so that those nominated to do the unsavoury task of looking after the vulnerable become the scapegoats for their suffering and demise.

The refusal to listen, to witness trauma narratives and other disturbing revelations in ways that allow them to be elaborated rather than shut down, is sometimes deliberate and sometimes due to defensive processes that are best described as unconscious. When deliberate, they are effective ways of perpetuating the trauma and abuse. When unconscious, they function to protect the individual witness to the testimony, or the community or society at large, from the disturbing import of what is being described. The unconscious temptation from which everyone suffers is the "going astray" that Laplanche (1999) describes—that we turn away from the things we know will make our lives harder to live; that every time we come up against something genuinely disturbing, we must fight an urge to go in a different direction, less troubling and threatening to our sense of stability. This is not necessarily morally culpable; people need to protect themselves from harm and the stakes can be very high. But when it comes to psychosocial violence such as is found in child abuse, the kind of silencing that comes about as a consequence of such defensive manoeuvres results in the sorts of repetitions that I have described above: hauntings of the present by events that should be in the past, but are continuously returning in old–new forms, trying to speak in ways that will enable them to be heard. Asserting that the general problem of witnessing trauma is the difficulty that victims have of *speaking* is one way of silencing them; it is more productive and more accurate to consider how the difficulty is really one of *listening*, and to notice how so much of our response to trauma narratives such as disclosures of sexual abuse is to create processes and structures that ensure that nothing happens. After such non-performative action, who can blame people if they no longer feel they should talk?

References

Ahmed, S. (2021). *Complaint!* London: Duke University Press.

Butler, J. (1997). *Excitable Speech: A Politics of the Performative*. London: Taylor & Francis.

Caruth, C. (1996). *Unclaimed Experience: Trauma, Narrative and History*. London: Johns Hopkins University Press.

Cesarani, D., & Levine, P. (2002). *Bystanders to the Holocaust: A Re-evaluation*. London: Routledge.

Felman, S. (1992). Education and crisis. In: S. Felman & D. Laub (Eds.), *Testimony: Crises of Witnessing in Literature, Psychoanalysis, and History*. New York: Routledge.

Ferenczi, S. (1949). Confusion of the tongues between the adults and the child (the language of tenderness and of passion). *International Journal of Psychoanalysis, 30*: 225–230.

Freud, S. (1909b). Analysis of a phobia in a five-year-old boy. *S. E., 10*: 1–150. London: Hogarth.

Frosh, S. (2013). *Hauntings: Psychoanalysis and Ghostly Transmissions*. London: Palgrave.

Frosh, S. (2019). The unsaid and the unheard. In: A. Murray & K. Durrheim (Eds.), *Qualitative Studies of Silence: The Unsaid as Social Action*. Cambridge: Cambridge University Press.

Glaser, D., & Frosh, S. (1988). *Child Sexual Abuse*. London: BASW/Macmillan.

Gordon, A. (1997). *Ghostly Matters: Haunting and the Sociological Imagination*. Minneapolis, MN: University of Minnesota Press.

Hlavka, H., & Mulla, S. (2021). *Bodies in Evidence: Race, Gender, and Science in Sexual Assault Adjudication*. New York: New York University Press.

Laplanche, J. (1999). The unfinished Copernican Revolution. In: J. Laplanche, *Essays on Otherness*. London: Routledge.

Laub, D. (1992). Bearing witness, or the vicissitudes of listening. In: S. Felman & D. Laub (Eds.), *Testimony: Crises of Witnessing in Literature, Psychoanalysis, and History*. New York: Routledge.

Levi, P. (1947). *If This Is a Man*. In: P. Levi, *If This Is a Man* and *The Truce*. London: Penguin, 1987.

Loewald, H. (1960). On the therapeutic action of psychoanalysis: In: H. Loewald, *Papers on Psychoanalysis*. New Haven, CT: Yale University Press, 1980.

Rothberg, M. (2019). *The Implicated Subject: Beyond Victims and Perpetrators*. Stanford, CA: Stanford University Press.

SHaME (Sexual Harms and Medical Encounters Project). (2021). Sexual Violence, Medicine, and Psychiatry Symposium, May 2021. https://shame.bbk.ac.uk/events/sexual-violence-medicine-and-psychiatry-symposium/

Shoesmith, S. (2016). *Learning from Baby P: The Politics of Blame, Fear, and Denial*. London: Jessica Kingsley.

Winnicott, D. W. (1969). The use of an object. *International Journal of Psychoanalysis, 50*: 711–716.

CHAPTER 4

Racial massacres and silencing in the American southern states

Roger Frie

Introduction

Several years ago, I was invited to give a lecture in New York on the theme of silencing and responsibility. As a practising psychoanalyst, who is also a historian and social philosopher, I am interested in how societies and individuals seek to silence mass racial violence and genocide. What are the social and psychological processes that enable responsibility for these grievous crimes to be kept at a distance? In turn, how might unacknowledged historical trauma affect the descendants of victims and perpetrators? My interest in this field stems from my therapeutic work with descendants of Holocaust survivors, and from the question of what it means to be a third-generation German whose own family members were supporters of the Third Reich. In my lecture, I recounted how my German family, like so many others in the post-war decades, remained silent about its Nazi past and sought to keep the Holocaust at bay (Frie, 2017, 2019). Yet as psychoanalysis teaches us, historical traumas do not disappear. They keep showing up, reminding us of their presence. Once we are ready to acknowledge the crimes of the past, we need to attend to the question of historical responsibility;

in essence, to learn how to fill the silence with words and begin an ethical dialogue. None of this is easy of course, and the process of reconciliation is never-ending. We cannot erase what was done, or hope to resolve it in the present. But I believe that the process of attending to the silences we encounter, and of listening to voices that have remained unheard, can offer us a pathway forward.

After I finished my lecture, I was approached by a white man with a notable southern American accent. He said that the process I discussed was familiar to him and that he had a history he wanted to share. My curiosity was piqued, and we arranged to meet. It was to be the first of many meetings that eventually led me to travel to America's Deep South and to visit an isolated area of the Mississippi River Delta, which is the site of one of the worst and least known racial massacres in United States history. It is called the Elaine Massacre and is located in Phillips County, Arkansas. It took place in 1919 and I travelled there exactly 100 years after the massacre began.

Today, the racial traumas of the past continue to shape American race relations and racial injustice in the present, not only in Elaine and the surrounding area but more generally. As a nation, the United States struggles to openly address its dark history of racial violence. Little I had seen or done until that point prepared me for what I found in Elaine, and yet the social and psychological dynamics I encountered there as I viewed the killing fields and spoke with descendants of the victims and perpetrators were familiar to me. In my discussion of the Elaine Massacre, I will focus on how the silence of the perpetrators has made it difficult for the victims to speak out, and on how the silence of the present continues to result in a silencing of the past (Frosh, 2019). It will be important to consider the different kinds of silence at work among the descendants of the victims and perpetrators and to examine the processes by which these silences have been maintained for over a century. Above all, I will suggest that the massacre and its effects show us how the drive to maintain white supremacy continues to shape American society today.

The Elaine Massacre

The town of Elaine is situated on the Mississippi River in the state of Arkansas. It sits opposite the state of Mississippi, to which it is connected by its long history of cotton growing, slavery, sharecropping, and white supremacy. Readers may recognise Arkansas as the state where President Bill Clinton grew up and where he later became governor. Another American icon, Elvis Presley, lived first in Mississippi and then in the city of Memphis, Tennessee, only several hours' distance from Elaine. Readers who are knowledgeable in American Blues music may be familiar with the city of Helena, Arkansas, which played a central role in its growth during the 1920s and 1930s. Helena was the location in which the Elaine Massacre was organised and where most of the perpetrators lived. It was also the city in which the southern man who approached me after my lecture, grew up.

David Solomon was nearly seventy when he first heard about the massacre. His father, who was nearly 100 years old, revealed that David's grandfather, a member of the white establishment, had provided support for the perpetrators who committed the crimes. David struggled to understand how it was that he had lived so much of his life without knowing about the massacre. He wondered whether it was similar for members of the African American community and approached a black man from Helena of a similar age. This man revealed to David that he had heard whispers of the massacre growing up, but only recently learned more about it. As David recounted:

> I asked him if he knew about the massacre. He said yes and we talked about it. He ended the conversation by observing that both the blacks and whites had kicked the event under the rug for so long that both continually tripped over it. This is as practical an explanation as I have ever heard for the presence of multigenerational trauma as well as for the palpable distrust between the communities that has lasted for 100 years. (David Solomon, personal communication)

The image of tripping over the rug is a good metaphor for what happens when perpetrator societies fail to address the historical trauma in their midst. The Elaine Massacre is an essential part of the fraught history of race relations in the United States. So long as these trauma-filled silences exist, it is difficult to imagine a path towards reconciliation and repair.

In the course of my research, I had the opportunity to speak with Sheila Walker on numerous occasions before she passed away in 2021. She was a direct descendant of the massacre's victims. Sheila welcomed the opportunity to tell me her family's story but began by sharing how she became aware of racism as a child. Sheila recalled that she was still very young and living in Chicago when her mother attended the funeral of fourteen-year-old Emmit Till, who had been horrifically murdered by white men in an act of racial terror. In the summer of 1955, Emmit had travelled from his home in Chicago to visit relatives near the small town of Money, Mississippi. During his stay, he was accused of offending a white woman at a local grocery store, which in the South was the most common trope used to justify the lynching of black men and boys. Emmit was abducted, beaten, and mutilated before he was shot, and his lifeless body was submerged in a river. His murderers were eventually arrested but found not guilty by an all-white jury. They escaped conviction even after admitting their crimes to the press the following year.

Emmit's mother, Meg Till, insisted that her son's mutilated body be seen. It lay in an open casket for three days, where it was seen by thousands who filed by in a solemn process of remembrance and acknowledgement. Emmit's murder and its aftermath exposed the culture of lynching and the depth of racial violence in the United States. It also demonstrated the limits of the democratic process at a time when African American life in southern states was governed by a racist system of Jim Crow laws.

Although she was still a young girl, Sheila said she clearly remembered the effect that attending Emmit's funeral had on her mother. When her mother came home that day, she took her daughters in her arms. Sheila recounted that "She held us tightly and wept." It was while being embraced, Walker said, that "I remember looking down at my left hand and thinking that just because of my skin colour, I could also be killed. It was at that moment that I first began to grasp how racism affected me." It is a moment she never forgot, one that continued to resonate for her. Sheila said that the current climate of racial hostility and violence in the United States reminded her of the kind of tensions that were evident so many decades ago when Emmit was viciously murdered. In fact, not only is this history of racial violence still present, it has also reverberated through Sheila's family over time. Indeed, what Sheila did not know as a young girl and learned only much later in life, was that her family members were survivors of the Elaine Massacre. The traumas they experienced shaped the trajectory of Sheila's family.

The conflagration

Since the Elaine Massacre is little known, I will begin with a descriptive account of violence and its root causes. The entry of the United States into the First World War was seen by many African Americans as an opportunity to increase their political rights. But any hopes that fighting for their country in the war might result in change when they returned home were quickly dashed (see Williams, 2010). White Americans feared that returning black soldiers could use their military training to demand equality and better labour conditions. Southern landowners were particularly fearful of black attempts to unionise to receive equal pay for the cotton they harvested in addition to fair wages for their labour. The white authorities used lynching and racial terror to assert absolute control and maximise their profits. In the summer and fall of 1919, vicious anti-black race riots erupted in twenty-six cities throughout the country. The worst violence occurred in Elaine, Arkansas.[1] The hatred and barbarity in evidence make for difficult reading.

When African American soldiers returned from the war, they joined with sharecroppers and began to unionise. They could not have imagined the kind of backlash they would face. The massacre began on the night of September 30, 1919, when a union meeting was called at the Hoop Spur church.[2] Black families gathered to hear speeches. Knowing of the threat posed by landowners, they posted guards outside to watch for trouble. Sheila Walker's great-grandmother, Sallie Giles, her teenage grandmother, Annie, and her two great-uncles, Milligan and Albert were among those in attendance. Gunfire suddenly broke out as white men working on behalf of the landowners peppered the church with bullets. Shots were returned by the black guards.

In the melee, a white man was killed. News of the killing travelled fast. In the dead of night, the Phillips County sheriff organised a posse of white men. Early on the morning of October 1, the men arrived at the church and the indiscriminate shooting of black people began.

---

[1] My account of the historical details of the Elaine Massacre draws chiefly on the following works of history: McWhirter, 2011; Stockley, 2001; Whitaker, 2008; Woodruff, 2003.

[2] A spur is a section of railway that usually extends off a main railroad track to allow for the loading and unloading of train cars.

Sharecroppers were murdered in the fields, in their homes, or as they ran for cover. Sallie and Annie hid in fear for their lives as they witnessed the killings. Milligan, who was only fifteen, was shot in the face and the bullet lodged in the back of his neck. Albert, the older brother, was pursued and shot five times. One of the bullets went through his skull.

Newspaper headlines and telegrams across the region spoke of a "Negro Uprising", fanning the flames of white hatred and insecurity. As the day progressed, armed white men from nearby towns and counties and the neighbouring states of Mississippi and Tennessee poured into the area, ready to unleash "white justice". As the armed white mob began to drive south on the road from Helena to Elaine, they shot men, women, and children in the fields where they worked. According to a *Memphis Press* reporter who travelled with one group, the fields were soon emptied, and men began shooting at the dead bodies that now littered the edge of the road, using them as target practice to unleash their rage (for a detailed account, see Whitaker, 2008).

At noon on October 1, the mayor of Elaine contacted the Arkansas governor, Charles Brough, to request the federal army. Brough wasted no time in sending a telegram to the US war secretary: "Race riots in Elaine, Phillips County, this state. Four white said to be killed. Negroes were said to be massing for an attack. Request commanding general Camp Pike be authorized to send such United States troops as may be necessary and called for by me" (quoted in Stockley, 2001, p. 3). Brough's request was immediately granted and on October 2, 600 federal troops entered Elaine. Many of the soldiers were battle-hardened and had just returned from Europe. Among their number was a twelve-gun machine-gun battalion that had only recently fought against the Germans on the Western Front.

Descent into barbarism

The military commander, Colonel Jenks, set up machine-gun posts and ordered his troops to shoot any blacks that refused to disarm or who were believed to be a threat. The killings and barbarities that began with the white mob on October 1 were now overtaken by the military. Soldiers were sent out to search the fields. In one instance a squad of soldiers surrounded some fifty blacks hiding in a bayou and opened fire.

Afterwards, only fifteen were reported arrested. In another instance, four black men were seen trying to move towards the river and were shot down by a machine gun. When the bodies were found, two of their number turned out to be black veterans who were still wearing their US army uniforms. The white soldiers whom they had fought alongside against a common enemy now turned their guns on them (see Whitaker, 2008, p. 122).

Troops were also sent to the large Lambrook plantation. While some soldiers shot at sharecroppers, others took the lead in interrogations. In his autobiography, *All Out of Step*, the white plantation owner and heir to the Listerine fortune, Gerard Lambert (1956), recounts that the military's interrogation of a black union leader devolved into torture, then murder. Lambert's racist outlook is evident in the account he provides:

> Troopers brought him to our company store and tied him with a stout cord to one of the wooden columns on the outer porch. He had been extremely insolent, and the troopers, stung by the loss of two of their men that day in the woods, had pressed him with questions. He continued his arrogance, and one white man, hoping to make him speak up, poured a can of kerosene over him. As he was unwilling to talk, a man suddenly tossed a lighted match at him. The coloured man went up like a torch and, in a moment of supreme agony, burst his bounds. Before he could get but a few feet he was riddled with bullets. The superintendent told me with some pleasure that they had to use a fire hose to put him out. (Lambert, 1956, p. 77)

Nor was this kind of barbarism isolated in nature. In 1925, a white Arkansas itinerant journalist, Sharpe Dunaway, wrote a book called *What a Preacher Saw Through a Keyhole in Arkansas*, for which he interviewed witnesses of the massacre. Although Dunaway was a racist, he wrote with clear aversion about troops that went on a "march of death" and "committed one murder after another with all the calm and deliberation in the world" (quoted in Whitaker, 2008, p. 118). There were almost 600 all-white troops involved, so it is unlikely that the entire military participated in the massacre, and more likely that certain units committed atrocities. Of the nearly 600 soldiers, some tended to injured sharecroppers like Milligan and Albert Giles, enabling them to survive. But the racism embedded in much of the military led to widespread atrocities, lynching, and torture (see Stockley, 2001; Whitaker, 2008). And indeed, in 1927, Bessie Ferguson, author of a pro-planter master's degree thesis about the massacre, wrote that barbarous acts such as "cutting off the ears or toes of dead negroes for souvenirs and the dragging of their bodies through the streets of Elaine are told by witnesses" (quoted in Woodruff, 2003, p. 87).

The horrific violence in Elaine was not an isolated act. From the late nineteenth century to the mid-twentieth century, white southern power used lynching as a primary tool to instil fear and terror. Lynching in the South took the form of extreme brutality: murderous acts of bodily mutilation, decapitation, burning, and torture. Over time, it became an accepted part of the culture of southern white supremacy. The harvesting of body parts as souvenirs is possibly the most gruesome aspect of this history. Yet as disturbing as it might seem, it was not uncommon. As Sherrilyn Ifill, who has researched the history of lynching and its effects points out, body parts (particularly fingers) were often kept in bottles and displayed in white homes. The viewing of such relics permitted a great many southern white Americans to have an awareness of lynching, even if they did not see the actual lynching itself (Ifill, 2018, p. 60)

Lynchings were often celebrated in public, festive occasions that drew large crowds of spectators who would have their photos taken with mutilated corpses, the smiling face of white men and boys juxtaposed with brutally murdered African Americans.[3] Historical evidence, often in the form of photographs, shows that children and entire families were

---

[3] https://lynchinginamerica.eji.org/report/. The southern states that are included in this study are: Alabama, Arkansas, Florida, Georgia, Kentucky, Louisiana, Mississippi, North Carolina, South Carolina, Tennessee, Texas, and Virginia. EJI also points out that during this period, in addition to the 4,084 lynchings in the South, a further 341 lynchings occurred chiefly in the following states: Illinois, Indiana, Kansas, Maryland, Missouri, Ohio, Oklahoma, and West Virginia. The lower numbers of lynchings in these states reflected to some degree the lower number of African Americans living there, and the fact that those states were not shaped by the same legacy of racial slavery. But according to EJI, those lynchings nevertheless shared many of the same gruesome characteristics.

frequently present at lynchings. The presence of children, who were not only excited observers but, in some cases even acted as torturers, ensured the continuation of the violent hatred and barbarities across generations. Documented lynching continued well into the mid-twentieth century, which means that there are still white adults alive today who witnessed lynching as children and carry these memories with them into the present (Ifill, 2018). According to the Equal Justice Initiative (2017), between 1877 and 1950 there were a total of 4,084 lynchings in the American South. Phillips County, Arkansas, where Helena and Elaine are located, has the ignominious distinction of having the highest recorded number of lynchings of all the southern counties.[4]

Anti-black violence came to a head during the Elaine Massacre. Most of the murders took place during the first three days. The final murder connected to the massacre occurred on October 7. On the same day, speaking on behalf of the landowners, Colonel Jenks issued a public announcement to sharecroppers to get them to return to the fields and harvest the cotton: "No innocent Negro has been arrested … All you have to do is remain at work just as if nothing had happened. Phillips county has always been a peaceful, law-abiding community, and normal conditions must be restored right away. Stop talking! Stay at home—Go to work—don't worry!" (quoted in Stockley, 2001, p. 81). On October 10, 1919, Arkansas governor, Charles Brough, wrote a personal note of thanks to the Secretary of War in Washington: "I am gratified to be able to inform you, Mr Secretary, that the white citizens of Phillips County … co-operated to the fullest extent to prevent mob violence, and at the same time run down bad negroes who were responsible for the outbreak" (quoted in Desmarais, 1974, p. 189).

The exact number of dead is unknown since there was no official count. Dunaway offered an unsubstantiated estimate of "856 … killed." (Dunaway, 1925, p. 109). Recently, the Equal Justice Initiative, which works towards racial reconciliation, has concluded that there were at least 234 dead. What is not in doubt is that after all the vicious, wanton

---

[4] According to EJI, there were at least 245 lynchings recorded in Phillips County during this period. EJI refers to the murder of African Americans in the Elaine Massacre as lynchings. As I will discuss below, the exact number of those killed in the massacre has long been a point of discussion, since exact figures remain unknown.

violence, not a single white was ever brought to trial. To this day, no official government investigation of the massacre has ever been carried out and it continues to be little known. What happened in Elaine reflects the United States as a whole. By 1960, nearly 5,000 lynchings had occurred yet not a single white person was ever brought to justice for the heinous crimes they committed (Ifill, 2018, p. 75).

The rule of silence

The silence that ensued after the massacre was like an icy blanket of snow and ice that refused to melt. It was the silence of white complicity encompassing not just Phillips County, but the state of Arkansas and its southern neighbours. It was a national silence, seemingly borne without shame. In Phillips County the status quo of white supremacy continued, unabated, spurred on by the false narrative that an attempted black uprising had been heroically quelled and cost the lives of five brave white men.

This narrative was supported by a steady string of reports that were issued from Helena. On October 3, *The Gazette*, Arkansas's leading newspaper, baldly stated that "Negroes Plan to Kill All Whites". On October 6, *The New York Times* ran a front-page article with the headline: "Planned Massacre of Whites Today: Negroes Seized in Arkansas Riots Confess to Widespread Plot".[5] These reports were aimed at fanning white fears and rage about the danger posed by African Americans—a racist trope that is still used to this day.

Many whites felt neither guilt nor shame, and those who did hid their participation. After the massacre, the whites of Helena proclaimed that Phillips County had never had a lynching and never would (Stockley, 2001). Yet in the years after the massacre, more black men were brutally lynched in Phillips County and their bodies were set aflame in front of crowds of onlookers. The capacity to deny the reality of racism has remained a feature of white American society, particularly in the rural South.

---

[5] *The New York Times Index, October-November-December, 1919*, Volume 7, No. 4 (p. 261).

The causes for white silence are complex and many-sided. The high number of churches throughout the towns of the rural South points to the fact that white (and black) communities perceived themselves as Christian. Yet in white churches, silence ruled; there was no acknowledgement at Sunday morning church services of the lynchings that occurred, even though racial violence was commonplace and common knowledge. In many communities, the history of lynching and the deep-seated racial hatred that gave way to gleeful expressions of violent rage existed side-by-side with Christian piety.

The whites didn't see or talk about the need for justice. By remaining silent, members of the white community who were not directly involved in the massacre became passively complicit in it. This complicity is widespread and continues to this day in white communities that either struggle or altogether refuse to acknowledge lynchings, mark their locations, or confront their responsibility for what took place. As a result, the socio-economic and psychological effects of this traumatic violence have lasted into the present and nourished a deep and abiding mistrust felt by many black communities towards their white neighbours.

The silence of the perpetrators reinforced the silencing of the victims. In the black community, there were fearful whispers, but the silence was essential to ensure safety. The African American writer, Richard Wright, lived in Elaine with his mother and brother in the years directly before the massacre occurred. What he saw and experienced there as a young boy in the year 1916 speaks to the level of vicious racial violence that thrived in the area and foreshadowed the horrors to come. In Elaine, Wright lived with his mother's aunt, Maggie, and her husband, Silas Hoskins. Wright's uncle ran a successful business in the town. The notion that a black man could run a business in a southern white town created deep resentment among whites because it ran up against their racial beliefs. It was this hatred and resentment that led to Silas Hoskins's lynching.

The young Wright, who was eight years old at the time, was forced to flee Elaine with his family members. But what he witnessed marked him for the remainder of his life. In 1945 Wright published his famous memoir, *Black Boy*, which gave an account of the racism he saw and experienced growing up in the Jim Crow South. In *Black Boy*, Wright recounted the painful aftermath of the lynching:

> Uncle Silas had simply been plucked from our midst and we, figuratively, had fallen on our faces to avoid looking at the white-hot face of terror that we knew loomed somewhere above us. This was as close as the white terror had ever come to me, and my mind reeled. Why had we not fought back, I asked my mother, and the fear that was in her made her slap me into silence. (Wright, 1945, p. 64)

The lynching of Silas Hoskins went unreported and unpunished and as the painful reaction of Wright's mother demonstrated, the silence was essential if they hoped to survive.

The kind of fear experienced by Wright's mother was widespread in the aftermath of the massacre. Those who were able to moved away. Yet stories of the massacre never entirely disappeared and continued to be shared between family members over time, cautionary tales, half-spoken and halting. Memory fragments that were passed down from one generation to the next. One black descendant who lives in Helena today is Brian Miller, who is a federal district court judge. His father was Helena's first black mayor. Growing up, Brian knew nothing about the massacre or the deaths of his four great-uncles. He first learned of what happened later in life, when he saw his father become visibly upset while reading an article in the *Arkansas Gazette* that described a riot that took place long ago. When Brian asked his father what the matter was, his father responded: "My uncles died. There's more to it than just this" (quoted in Clancy, 2019). Miller's father was reticent to say more, so Brian needed to ask other family members before he could fill in the blanks. The silence he encountered was not unusual, even many decades later. As Brian says, "It was an ugly part of our history and it was something that most people didn't want to remember" (quoted in Clancy, 2019). He has described the scattering of his family that followed the massacre:

> Four of our great uncles were killed in the massacre. Our great-grandmother, Eliza Miller was called to identify the bodies. Our great-aunt Mariah Miller-Johnston identified the cold body of her husband, David Augustine Johnston, with horror. She immediately left Phillips County and never returned … Our great-uncle Lucien Miller moved to Chicago and never returned. Our great-aunt, Katie Miller moved to Los Angeles

and rarely returned. Our grandfather, Robert Miller, was only 13. Eliza [his mother] was so grief-stricken at what she witnessed and horrified at the thought of her youngest son being killed, that she packed him up and sent him away. My grandfather grew up isolated from his family in Boston. This had a profound effect on him, and later on his relationships with our father, Robert Miller Jr., our Aunt Maxine, and our Aunt Doris. My grandfather's journey as a result of the massacre had some effects on my family that are too painful to discuss. (Miller, 2019)

Miller says that now that he knows the history and the events of the massacre, he can "understand how [his grandfather] was shaped ... It created a detachment that had a ripple effect on our family for years to come" (quoted in Clancy, 2019).

The trauma endured by Sheila Walker's family as a result of the massacre led them to move first to a distant town in Arkansas, where Sheila was born, and then on to Chicago. When Sheila was a child, she often visited her uncle Jim, whom she remembers fondly as a kind and gentle man. It was only decades later that she learned that Uncle Jim, as she knew him, was Milligan Giles, the fifteen-year-old boy who almost died in the massacre. After being arrested, Milligan had been given a sentence of twenty-one years, but he was eventually released. Her other great-uncle, Albert, was given a death sentence that was ultimately commuted, but he was scarred for life.

Sheila first learned that something terrible had happened when she was in her twenties. It was the early 1970s and she was visiting her grandmother, Annie Giles, in Arkansas. In the course of spending time together, her grandmother shared stories of the past. As Sheila told me, Annie began to describe events that happened to her when she was a teenager. She recounted going to the Hoop Spur church with her mother and brothers to attend a union meeting. According to Sheila, there was a quiver in Annie's voice as she said: "I knew that something was going to happen in that church—and then they started shooting. People were dying in front of me. I grabbed some children and got out of the church through the back." Reliving this memory caused Annie to collapse in tears and she was unable to finish the story. After that, each time Sheila visited, she asked her grandmother what happened, and each time Annie would break down, unable to continue. It was not until many years later, in the 1990s, that Sheila's mother helped her to understand what Annie had said. She suggested that Annie might be referring to the "Elaine Riot". Sheila's mother must have had a sense of what happened but had refrained from speaking about it with her daughter. The silence of each generation had successively shaped the next.

Psychoanalysis suggests that the transmission of memory often includes unsaid and unresolved experiences of trauma. This is what the French psychoanalyst, Nicolas Abraham, once described as "the gaps left within us by the secrets of others" (Abraham, 1994, p. 171). Intergenerational secrets may be sensed long before they are consciously known. Traumatic histories are transmitted from one generation to the next, their meanings implicitly communicated in codes of silence, or more directly through the emotional experience of one's elders, conveying a message of what may or may not be talked about. The survivors of the massacre, along with their descendants, had powerful reasons for remaining silent. But the rule of silence among the perpetrators and bystanders was, if anything, even stronger. After the massacre, white residents of Phillips County did not talk about what happened. Their silence encompassed churches, newspapers, schools, and the judicial system. It is a silence that still exists today and has been difficult to break.

Silent complicity

About 500 people are living in the town of Elaine today. Many of the buildings on Main Street, where the white mob and the army once gathered, are almost empty. Some storefronts are shuttered, and others sit in a dilapidated state. The atmosphere can feel stifling and ominous. The presence of many confederate flags, which in recent years have become associated with the extreme right wing in the United States, made it easy to empathise with the unease experienced in the black community. The wealth divide between black and white mirrors the long history of injustices (see Stoppford, 2020). In rural towns like Elaine, 65 per cent of African Americans live below the poverty line, compared to just 13 per cent of whites. The black community lives on one side of town and the white community on the other. Schools remain segregated in all but name. Public schools are almost all black while most white children attend private academies.

When you are somewhere unfamiliar it's easy to misinterpret what you see and hear. The rural South is a place that is often misunderstood. Its horrifically violent history and continuing racial tensions loom large in the minds of visitors. Yet I couldn't overcome the disquiet I felt as I walked Elaine's streets and tried to imagine what it may have been like to live there 100 years ago. The denial and wilful disregard shown by many whites towards the history of the massacre illustrates just how hard it is to work towards acknowledgement and reconciliation. For example, Elaine's hardware store owner questions the high death toll and wonders how events that took place 100 years ago can still be relevant (Edwards, 2018). Similarly, Elaine's former mayor believes that the discussion of a massacre is "somebody trying to make something out of nothing much to talk about" (quoted in Nasir, 2019). While acknowledging that violence took place, the former mayor doubts its effects and the levels of violence that have been cited. Many in the white community deny the facts of history or continue to insist it remains irrelevant.

Sherrilyn Ifill helps us to understand the reactions of whites, above their insistence on remaining silent. According to Ifill, the silence that has accompanied the long history of lynching is powerful and hard to break:

> Whites do not talk about historical incidents of racial violence even among themselves. The reasons for maintaining the silence are plentiful. Some whites simply do not regard these incidents as having continuing relevance in the 21st century. For them, discussing lynching is merely an exercise in dredging up the past, and an unpleasant past. Other whites may fear that breaking the silence on these violent events will place them on the defensive, the blacks will be accusatory and will try to compel whites to take responsibility for actions that many will claim they knew nothing about. The more complex issue of what it means to be a beneficiary of a violent oppressive regime may remain unexplored as white participants insist on their innocence. For racial crimes for which perpetrators may still be alive, whites may fear that they will be called as witnesses in a reopened investigation or prosecution of an elderly perpetrator ... Even more complicated is the discovery by young family members of the

complicity of their parents and grandparents in violent racial oppression. Whites may find themselves deeply conflicted by the realization that family members were Klansmen, present at lynchings or deeply implicated in racial murder or assault. (Ifill, 2018, pp. 134–135)

As Ifill notes, opening up the history of racial violence to scrutiny can result in the painful recognition of the role played by one's family members in the horrors that were committed and subsequently silenced. Indeed, as the dynamics of post-war German memory suggest (Frie, 2017, 2019), the need to dissociate and remain silent about shameful perpetrator histories in one's own family and the immediate community continues to be strong, despite the passage of time. Certainly, the silence that exists among perpetrator groups is complex and many-sided. It can also be variously motivated. What interests me is how silence is maintained over time. Except for select members of the white community, silence regarding the historical facts of the Elaine Massacre, and acknowledgement and responsibility for what took place, have remained normative in and around Elaine. This silence has continued to exist despite broader shifts in American society, be it as a result of the civil rights movement or the very slow, but incremental change in how the white and black communities interact with one another, even in the Deep South. The example of Elaine suggests that broader societal shifts have not resulted in a concomitant willingness to address the dark past on a local level. This is also why Ifill insists that the work of recognition and reconciliation must occur at a local level.

Since family and community loom large, what role do they play in the maintenance of silence and the construction of memory? Contemporary narrative and memory studies (Brockmeier, 2018) suggest that individual understanding of the past is generated by our social interactions and our cultural contexts. Differently put, our relationships with other people create the conditions for what is said or not said, for which stories are told and which have yet to be heard. Viewed from afar, we might justifiably wonder how it is that descendants of perpetrator groups do not know about the crimes committed by their forbears. However, when considered from the perspective of the social dynamics of silencing and the construction of memory, the question,

"How could they not know?" is inherently limited. A better question might be: "What would knowing about the massacre and a familial connection to it mean?" By posing this kind of question, I am suggesting that we should look for complexity and avoid drawing a simple line between knowing and not knowing, or between silence and speaking out about the massacre and its consequences.

Another way of thinking about the process I am describing is to adopt a hermeneutic viewpoint, which allows us to reflect on our situatedness. What does it mean to be situated in a family and community that actively seeks to keep the past at bay, and that silences any talk of acknowledgement or responsibility? When a person is situated in a context that is shaped by silencing, then their awareness, or what a hermeneuticist might call their "world horizon", is necessarily limited. I am not suggesting that we should excuse ignorance or a stance that wilfully ignores historical facts. Rather, I am pointing to the process of social interaction through which boundaries are created and maintained. These boundaries, in turn, shape and limit what we know, understand, or can talk about at any point in time. As a result of the silencing that takes place in social interaction, where some aspects of the past are talked about and others are covered over, certain experiences will remain outside our conscious awareness. This points us back to the nature of the unconscious. As the hermeneutic psychoanalyst, Philip Cushman has suggested, "The unconscious is not an interior thing, but part of the patient's social landscape that contains potential feelings, thoughts, and experiences that are not able to show up because they lie on the other side of the patient's horizon of understanding" (Cushman, 1995, p. 307).

To appreciate what it means to reach the other side of a "horizon of understanding", consider the social formation of memory. A memory may be beyond our grasp, not because it is lodged somewhere in the dark recesses of our mind, but because it never found its way into the social interactions that shape what we know, understand, and can talk about. Thus, when families and communities actively silence certain topics, these topics may effectively be kept out of conscious awareness. To put it very simply, memories can remain "unknown" until they have been articulated in communication with other people. As the American interpersonalist, Harry Stack Sullivan (1953) once observed: "One has information about one's experience only to the extent that one has tended to communicate it to another or thought about it in the manner of communicative speech. Much of what is ordinarily said to be repressed is merely unformulated" (p. 185).

Contesting the past

For African American community members, the silence of the white community is experienced not only as a form of complicity in what took place, but also as an active refusal to acknowledge what the black community has endured, and the kinds of racial discrimination they continue to struggle with in the present. After a century of silence and silencing, one wonders whether the process of remembering and working through can ever really take place. Breaking the silence to openly acknowledge the mass racial violence and remember the victims is difficult to do, especially in places like Phillips County, Arkansas. It disrupts the status quo. In many cases, the creation of memorials can play an important role in this process. But creating memorials for the victims of racial violence is challenging because of the historical white ownership of public spaces. Additionally, while a memorial might act as a tangible reminder that violence and criminality took place, it is at best an initial step in a process that must address not only the past but also the deep injustices and inequalities of the present.

It is thus significant to note that in September 2019, exactly 100 years after the catastrophe, a privately funded memorial to the victims of the Elaine Massacre was established in Helena. It was the first attempt to remember the massacre publicly and, notably, the memorial was privately funded by a group of prominent descendants of the victims and perpetrators, most of whom live outside the area. David Solomon, who approached me after my lecture in New York, played a central role in the memorial's creation. He was joined by other descendants of the perpetrators including Chester Johnson, and descendants of the victims, including Brian Miller and Sheila Walker, among others. Together, this group worked to create a dialogue that might fill the silence and spur the process of remembering and reconciliation (Johnson, 2020). But the memorialisation has been contested. Many of the region's white residents choose to ignore the memorial altogether, while many members of Elaine's African American community understandably argue that the money used for the memorial could have been better spent to address poverty and create educational opportunities.

The issue of education is important. The impulse to deny the history of racial violence is strong. In Arkansas, as elsewhere in the American South, Republican-controlled governments are actively creating laws that dictate what public schools can teach about racism and its vicious history. Attempts to legislate history are the latest in a long line of steps that seek to maintain the silence and ensure white supremacy. Not only has the Elaine Massacre been absent from local school curricula, and in the state as a whole, it has until now been absent from virtually all school curricula across the country. To be sure, there are also signs of change, as the Black Lives Matter movement in the wake of the murder of George Floyd in the summer of 2020 illustrates. But the challenges for remembering, reconciliation, and reparation are enormous. And so long as a white public is not educated about its dark history, the persistence of dehumanising attitudes will be allowed to fester.

Conclusion: a personal reflection

The work of remembering I have described has been largely social and communal in scope. But, of course, it also needs to be personal in nature. Thus, I want to conclude by considering how my discussion of the Elaine Massacre might relate to who I am. How does it reflect my location at the intersection of culture and history? I hope to encourage readers to similarly consider their positions. For a Canadian, the impulse to ignore what happens in the state of Arkansas is strong and, indeed, many white Canadians prefer to say that racism is something that occurs only south of the border, thereby effectively silencing Canada's dark history (Frie, 2020). Not only was Canada a slave-holding nation for more than 200 years, black Canadians today continue to suffer disproportionately from racism and systemic discriminatory practices.

The history of the black community in Canada mirrors the experience of Indigenous peoples. In the summer of 2021, approximately 1,000 unmarked graves of Indigenous children were discovered in western Canada, next to so-called Indian Residential Schools. Schools in name only, these were institutions of assimilation and genocide whose purpose was to extinguish Indigenous life and culture (Fontaine, Craft, and The Truth and Reconciliation Commission of Canada, 2015). Run chiefly by the Catholic Church and paid for by the Canadian government, the last of these schools were only shut down in 1996. The gruesome discovery of unmarked graves was "news" only to non-Indigenous Canadians, and in the coming years it is expected that many more unmarked graves will be found. For the past century, Indigenous people have been telling anyone who would listen that their children are missing. But the silence continued for so long because no one in the white authority structure was willing to listen or acknowledge what Indigenous leaders were saying. By silencing their voices, Canadian authorities hoped to suppress the history of the Indian Residential Schools and the horrors that occurred there.

Now that the dreadful history of Canada's Indian Residential Schools is being acknowledged, there is the possibility of starting a process of reconciliation. But even in the face of more open and honest discourse about the past, dissociation remains a powerful force if we are not ready or willing to grasp the meaning of what we learn. All of this has a particular resonance for me. I spent much of my childhood only one hour away from an Indian Residential School. Growing up, I was completely ignorant of its existence and the kind of horrors that took place there: sexual and physical abuse, starvation, disease, and death. How could I have not known? And now that I do know, how and what can I contribute to the process of reconciliation? What words do I find to fill the silence? Looking back, it seems that the story which the elderly southern gentleman first told me in New York is not so different from my own.

References

Abraham, N. (1994). Notes on the phantom: A complement to Freud's metapsychology. In: N. T. Rand (Ed.), *The Shell and the Kernel: Renewals of Psychoanalysis* (pp. 171–176). Chicago, IL: University of Chicago Press.

Brockmeier, J. (2018). *Beyond the Archive: Memory, Narrative, and the Autobiographical Process*. New York: Oxford University Press.

Clancy, S. (2019, September 29). Marking a tragedy: Memorial to those who died in the Elaine Massacre enmeshed in controversy. *Arkansas Democrat-Gazette*. Retrieved from https://arkansasonline.com

Cushman, P. (1995). *Constructing the Self, Constructing America: A Cultural History of Psychotherapy*. Cambridge, MA: Da Capo Press.

Desmarais, R. H. (1974). Military intelligence reports on Arkansas riots: 1919–1920. *Arkansas Historical Quarterly*, 33(2): 189–202.

Dunaway, L. S. (1925). *What a Preacher Saw Through a Keyhole in Arkansas*. Little Rock, AR: Parke-Harper.

Edwards, B. (2018, April 23). Divided town struggles to remember what happened during 1919 Arkansas killings. *Montgomery Advisor*. Retrieved from https://montgomeryadvertiser.com

Equal Justice Initiative (2017). *Lynching in America: Confronting the Legacy of Racial Terror* (3rd edn.). Montgomery, AL: Equal Justice Initiative.

Fontaine, P., Craft, A., & Truth and Reconciliation Commission of Canada (2015). *A Knock on the Door: The Essential History of Residential Schools from the Truth and Reconciliation Commission of Canada*. Winnipeg, MN: University of Manitoba Press.

Frie, R. (2017). *Not in My Family: German Memory and Responsibility After the Holocaust*. New York: Oxford University Press.

Frie, R. (2019). History's ethical demand: Memory, denial, and responsibility in the wake of the holocaust. *Psychoanalytic Dialogues*, 29(1): 122–142.

Frie, R. (2020). Recognizing white racism in Canada. *Psychoanalysis, Self, and Context*, 15(3): 276–280.

Frosh, S. (2019). The unsaid and the unheard: Acknowledgement, accountability, and recognition in the face of silence. In: A. J. Murray & K. Durrheim (Eds.), *Qualitative Studies of Silence: The Unsaid as Social Action* (pp. 254–269). Cambridge: Cambridge University Press.

Ifill, S. (2018). *On the Courthouse Lawn: Confronting the Legacy of Lynching in the 21st Century* (2nd edn.). Boston, MA: Beacon.

Johnson, C. (2020). *Damaged Heritage: The Elaine Race Massacre and a Story of Reconciliation*. New York: Pegasus.

Lambert, G. B. (1956). *All Out of Step: A Personal Chronicle*. Garden City, NY: Doubleday.

McWhirter, C. (2011). *Red Summer: The Summer of 1919 and the Awakening of Black America*. New York: Henry Holt.

Miller, B. (2019, August 24). Honor the dead, recognize massacre, heal division. *Arkansas Democrat Gazette*. Retrieved from https://www.arkansasonline.com

Nasir, N. (2019, July 25). In a small Arkansas town, echoes of a century-old massacre. *AP News*. Retrieved from https://apnews.com

Stockley, G. (2001). *Blood in Their Eyes: The Elaine Race Massacres of 1919*. Fayetteville, AR: University of Arkansas Press.

Stoppford, A. (2020). *Trauma and Repair: Confronting Segregation and Violence in America*. Lanham, MD: Rowman & Littlefield.

Sullivan, H. S. (1953). *Conceptions of Modern Psychiatry*. New York: W. W. Norton.

Whitaker, R. (2008). *On the Laps of Gods: The Red Summer of 1919 and the Struggle for Justice that Remade a Nation*. New York: Three Rivers.

Williams, C. L. (2010). *Torchbearers of Democracy: African-American Soldiers in the World War I Era*. Chapel Hill, NC: University of North Carolina Press.

Woodruff, N. E. (2003). *The American Congo: The African American Freedom Struggle in the Delta*. Cambridge, MA: Harvard University Press.

Wright, R. (1945). *Black Boy*. New York: Harper & Brothers.

CHAPTER 5

Silencing of female voices in medical history: the silenced girl who cried pain

Babette S. Gekeler

Introduction

Behind every statistic lie individual women's and girls' names and stories that collectively mirror the enhancing yet grim social reality revealing nearly two-thirds of the world's illiterate adults are women. Out of the 781 million adults over the age of fifteen estimated to be illiterate, 496 million were women, the World's Women 2015 report found. Women made up more than half the illiterate population in all regions of the world. The largest gaps are in South Asian areas where illiteracy rates are 23 per cent for men, but 42 per cent for women (United Nations, 2012). While every additional year of primary school auspiciously increases girls' eventual wages by 10–20 per cent and encourages them to marry later and have fewer children, leaving them less vulnerable to violence, global statistics show that just 39 per cent of rural girls attend secondary school, compared to 45 per cent of rural boys, 59 per cent of urban girls and 60 per cent of urban boys (UN Women, 2019).

Additionally, while in almost all countries acceptance of violence against women and girls had decreased over time, around one in three women have been the victim of physical or sexual violence—around two-thirds of them faced violence or death at the hand of an intimate partner or family member. The report found that around 60 per cent of all women survivors did not report the crime or seek support. Those who did turned to family or friends rather than the police (UN Women Data on Sexual Violence against Women and Girls, 2023).

These numerically summarised circumstances relate to an age-old pattern of women and their body representation in a historical biomedical rationale that claimed scientific proof of female inferiority, that prescribed "hysterical" patients the "rest cure", inherently perpetuating and anchoring women as weak and pathological. The functional underpinnings of the rationale justify sex discrimination by the ways women have been diagnosed, defined, and often silenced throughout society remain invariantly potent even today. Its vestiges are particularly evident in abortion policy and other reproductive rights struggles.

On June 24, 2022, the US Supreme Court overturned *Roe v. Wade*, the landmark piece of legislation that made access to abortion a federal right in the United States. The right-wing extremist Republican lobby and evangelical Christians fought for decades to scrap the 1973 ruling giving women the right to choose. President Trump's three appointees to the court, Justices Neil Gorsuch, Brett Kavanaugh, and Amy Coney Barrett, formed the backbone of the five to four majority that threw out past decisions upholding abortion rights. Kavanaugh and Barrett each replaced former justices—Anthony Kennedy and Ruth Bader Ginsburg, respectively—who had backed abortion rights. The public's voice pronounces this ruling as regressive, dangerous, and insulting since it dismantles legal protection and paves the way for individual states to curtail or outright ban abortion rights (American University Washington DC, 2022). Consequently, abortion rights are high on the political agenda and likely to be central in the autumn campaign and the 2024 presidential election.

Like fresh red blood lancing through the veins in an old leaf at a time when a critical mass of women came to understand that seeing and thinking for themselves was fundamental to their liberation, old flames light up in the collective minds of women. A time when feminists challenged an age-old, male-dominated medical establishment, that for centuries had clung to the idea that domesticity and motherhood, with their attributes of gentleness, submission, and self-sacrifice, were the best prerequisites for a woman's physical and mental health. Ambiguity and uncertainty accompany our modern times where binary under-pinnings of womanhood, as well as that of malehood in addition to all deliberations of gender forms, such as bi-, trans-, and asexuality, are being more contested than ever before. A time where social categories are being challenged and ruptured, fractured, re-imagined and recon-structed is a fragile time for all people in vulnerable social positions—women as much as children, ethnic and religious minorities, refugees, the mentally ill, the homeless, and so on. Exclusion via silencing is part of a much broader and more complex way that some cultures "think", in processes:

> whereby the human body, psychic forms, geographical space, and the social formation are all constructed within interrelating and dependent hierarchies of high and low (...) [as] a fundamental basis to mechanisms of ordering and sense-making in European cultures. (Stallybrass & White, 1986, pp. 2–3)

Grounding male hegemony in the fundamental kinkiness of woman-hood and the idea that the female body is inferior, defective, and always dependent on the whims of the womb led to the silencing and with-holding of information, constructing the needs of women according to the political and cultural interests at the correspondent times. While over time and through the ages, women have been doctors, counsel-lors, nurses, pharmacists, midwives, abortionists, sisters, and moth-ers—experts of their bodies and *wise women* in the vernacular—for the authorities, they were inapt, minor, witches, and quacks.

In order to shed light on the silencing of women, not only histori-cally but currently, particularly at times of crises, as well as the idea of "self-silencing" in their intimate participation within the therapeutic practice space—the following section will roughly trace some historical lines of how women were expected to think and feel about their bod-ies. Pursuantly, feminine identity formations had been forged along the conditions of historical representations of what constitutes a woman. The section will elucidate a deeply embodied paradox: that of femaleness and womanhood. This paradox corroborates the relentless inner conflict of being deeply enamoured yet abrasively appalled by the female body.

Pathological narratives and the silencing of women's experiences

The medical world is a powerful one, constructed in a conservative male voice, which encapsulates the silencing of female voices. Pathological narratives are built along imagery of the male body as a standard; thus, it has been argued to be deeply androcentric (Hibbs, 2014). The privileges of masculinity mirror the corresponding deprivileges of the feminine—like a figure-ground pattern of Gestalt psychology. From the first, the body of the female practitioner in medicine has been understood as incomplete, deficient, inadequate, intemperate, and unruly. Thus, it had to be kept contained in a "feminine" sphere, a sphere which maintained a belief that women's nerves are too fraught and frail to endure an education since her ovaries would get inflamed if she were to read (Cleghorn, 2021; Perkins Gilman, 2007).

According to Hippocrates of Kos—who is considered the father of medicine and who lived in the fifth and fourth centuries BC—illness was not a punishment of the gods but an imbalance within our human bodies. He invented the case historical method and swore to treat all illnesses of all humans to the best of his knowledge and belief. This oath is the earliest expression of medical ethics in the Western world, establishing several principles of medical ethics, including those of confidentiality and non-maleficence, which still remain of paramount significance (Cleghorn, 2021). Hippocrates acknowledged that women needed to be treated differently from males and require specific healing methods. However, his statement is historically embedded in a patriarchal age where women barely held civil and human rights, and girls belonged to their fathers and women to their husbands (ibid.). They owned no land or possessions and were not called to make autonomous choices over their bodies. They were seen as weaker, more indolent, and smaller versions of the male ideal. Insufficient and imperfect by way of being *different* from men. Particularly the uterus organ was a difference that made for a lasting myth about the female body. In ancient Greece, the belief circulated that the uterus possesses a hunger for sex and pregnancy that defies the control of the woman in whose body it rests. Additionally, it was believed to wander around the body harming those organs it would touch, and causing a plethora of symptoms, such as convulsions, epileptic seizures, hallucinations, dyspnoea, pain, and hemiplegia (Cleghorn, 2021). Such ideas are grounded in the masculine medical discourse on the subservience of women to the organ by which they were controlled. Thus, the symbolic nature of a being who is submissive, dependent, cryptic, and at someone else's mercy had been born and carries well into collective social representations of "woman" today.

The defectiveness of the female found its way into medieval European Christianity, which made the female responsible for all earthly sins. Eve, in the Book of Genesis, has been initially incomplete and imperfect as she sprang out of the ribs of Adam and brought only ruin based on her obstinacy and libidinousness. Women were now not only submissive and dependent but deviant. Medicine fell into the hands of Christian men, perpetuating the belief of the female body being a vessel of sin. Religious superstitions that saw illness as divine punishment mingled with medical prejudices about the destructive potential of women's bodies. *Fascination and fear* of the female body in light of the mysterious feminine biology led to cataclysmal consequences.

In the years 1346–1356 a large portion of the European population were killed by the Black Death (Cleghorn, 2021). This unprecedented epidemic had been of such force and scale that many believed it to be a punishment from God. The Church as well as society at large was in search of a scapegoat for this catastrophe and the costs of the decimation of the population. Accepted beliefs about women's dependence on men, their innate physical and mental weakness, and their unruly, uncontrollable organs and biological processes were sweetened with a new suspicion around women's deviant and demonic potential of being the architects of sin, working in the name of the devil. Heinrich Kramer, a passionate German Inquisitor, wrote the *Malleus Maleficarum* (The Hammer of Witches, published 1486 in the city of Speyer) explaining with passionate detail the existence of witches and witchcraft. For a woman to be infected with witchcraft, she must have one of three specific vices: infidelity, ambition, and lust. The more insatiable the woman, the more likely the devil is to take the form of an incubus and lie with her (Broedel, 2003). Any woman whose lifestyle, behaviour, and personality didn't conform to the highest virtues of chastity and faith became suspicious. Prevalent fears in a superstitious social climate in turn led women to easily fall under suspicion: "Any occurrence of an inexplicable event quickly became a threatening situation to those already vilified for being obstreperous, angry, deviant, solitary or strange" (Cleghorn, 2021, p. 49). In a complicated collusion of the religious, social, and political climate, during the sixteenth and seventeenth centuries approximately 50,000 people were executed for the crime of witchcraft, of whom 80 per cent were women, many over the age of forty (Kors & Peters, 2001; Levack, 2006). The last witch was burned in Europe in 1811.

An English physician and chemist named Edward Jordan wrote *A Brief Discourse of a Disease Called the Suffocation of the Mother*, in 1603, this being the first work in English on symptoms associated with the disorders of the uterus (*the Mother*). Hysteria would take its place as the all-encompassing medical model in the pursuing centuries (from Greek *hysteria* = uterus), pathologising the relationship between women's bodies and minds. In 1636, the book *The Sick Woman's Private Looking Glass* was published by the physician John Sadler, who claimed that via a lack of "Instruction", women suffer their pain since they are uneducated and demure. A woman's decency keeps the "ail" from being revealed to the doctor leading to her grief to secretly increase her ail. The ailment of women from having a uterus continued through the publications and writings of male physicians. In addition to physical ailments such as cramps, epilepsy, apoplexy, paralysis, dehydration, malignant ulcers, and other anomalies, the disastrous effect of the uterus on the nerves and the mind increasingly came to the fore. If the uterus is underused and left empty and inactive, women were at risk of going insane. Anatomist William Harvey suspected in 1651 that unnatural circumstances of the uterus would spawn mental symptoms of the "worst" kind (Cleghorn, 2021). Most physiological or mental symptoms which have supposedly been caused by a sickened or underused uterus were termed "hysteric" throughout the seventeenth century. The word denominated "relating to the uteri". "Hysteria has become the nosological grey area for all nameless women's diseases, which one must call mysteries given the innumerable disease states that cavort in the orbit of this term" (Weir Mitchell, 1875, p. 94). By the mid-seventeenth century, nearly all diseases befalling women were merged within a panacea defined as "hysteric passions". Everything from heart and breathing troubles, liver complaints, muscle weakness, and pregnancy complications to dizziness, weeping, laughing, absurd speech, and eye-rolling to customary chokings, fainting, convulsions, and contortions became hysteria (Willis, 1681). Well into the nineteenth century, when Jean-Martin Charcot, a leading neurologist at Paris's notorious Salpetriere Hospital asylum, was determined in the 1870s to solve the riddles continually surrounding hysteria, the mysterious ailment became a subject of the psychoanalytic gaze.

Sigmund Freud significantly contributed to the hardening inter-linking of hysteria as a mental illness and the construction of scientific knowledge in the silencing of women. His therapeutic project was the re-inflexion of this grotesque material into comic form. When his hysteric patient Emmy von N. (1895d, pp. 109–110) can look at the "grotesque figures" and "laugh without a trace of fear" it is as if Freud has managed a singular restitution, salvaging torn shreds of carnival from their phobic alienation in the bourgeois unconscious by making them once more the object of cathartic laughter, similar to the alleviation of the suffering of his equally recognised patient Anna O. Such carnival debris spills out of the mouths of those terrified Viennese women in Freud's *Studies on Hysteria* (Breuer & Freud, 1895d). Unmistakably, these phobia-producing masks, rituals, and symbols displayed at the carnivals are plundered with ethnographic material from alien, non-European cultures. "Clownism" as a photographic representation was frequently attested to as a symptomatic aspect of hysteria. Freud in a letter to Fliess (1954) refers to the "perversion of the seducers" (the patients themselves) who "connect up nursery games and sexual scenes", combining carnivalesque symptomatology to a purely sexual aetiology. In such a way socio-historical matrices of symptoms remain obscured and powerful images of the lesser woman and alien as the "low other" conjoined.

Carlo Bonomi (2017) profoundly delineates the castration complex and sees the most significant context for the trauma of castration in the genital mutilation of Freud's patient, Emma Eckstein. In line with the Victorian ethic of puritanism the widespread subjection of women to genital mutilation, circumcision, and castration as a medical treatment for masturbation, was prevalent in Freud's time. One such surgeon was Isaak Baker Brown, member of the Royal College of Surgeons and co-founder of St. Mary's Hospital in London, who published his book *On the Curability of Certain Forms of Insanity, Epilepsy, Catalepsy and Hysteria in Females* in 1866, where he ascribes a plethora of symptoms of hysteria all to the aetiology of an excited clitoris. Today's biological knowledge, of course, that an organ such as the clitoris consisting of around 8,000 nerves will be sensitive and in a swollen state, at Freud's time was seen as pathological and breaking the code of ethics of proper women, who were submitted to the most harrowing clitoridectomies. As Bonomi argues, resulting genital injury was neglected and repressed both in the analysis of Emma and in nineteenth- and early twentieth-century paediatrics leading to what he names an "unformulated trauma". Unformulated trauma, in turn, furthers both personal and social anxieties. In Bonomi's view, Freud's work on the biological speculation on the inherited nature of the unconscious memories of castration was the consequence of his active repression originating in the traumatic scene of genital mutilation.

While unformulated trauma creates a gap both on a symbolic and a concrete level following Freud's professional thinking for a long time, the problem of communication while there is a traumatic and repressed experience in the background was, according to Bonomi, perceived by Ferenczi who unconsciously tried to fill that gap by "expressing what had been muted in his master" (Gymesi, 2019), by giving a proper reaction to Emma Eckstein's cut: the recognition and acceptance of the true reason for the patient's suffering. In other words, the ending of the silencing of women's voices and experiences. In marking hysteria, a mental illness, hysteric women had gone from "having lost control, to being out of control, to being hyper-sexual, enthralled by fantasies, possessed and now mad. Unbuckled from the body, hysteria had become a cultural leitmotif for feminine temperament unbound, untamed, unbidden" (Cleghorn, 2021, p. 158).

The marriage of psychoanalysis and hysteria can be understood as the articulation and establishment of a system of understanding identity and subjectivity in which women are always constituted as the negated obverse of men (Devereux, 2014). By establishing an essentialised normality, any women's objection finds itself expressible only somatically, through the body. A condition that in the last decade of the nineteenth century became the redefined women's "disease" of hysteria. Thus, opposing of the patriarchal system by women was comprehensible as a pathology—and moreover, as Devereux (2014) suggests, a pathology without origin other than the fact of femininity.

Since hysteria has over the last decades been implicitly demoted to a broader, less specific category of disorder, it has lost its status as an identifiable clinical disorder. Critical feminist discourse identifies its historical link to femininity for hundreds of years. Yet, while there is a celebratory aspect to the continuous relegation of hysteria as a diagnosis, discourse insists that it is not to be understood solely as a medical condition but a cultural one, an embodied index of the forms of silencing. Showalter (1993, p. 286) describes it as "a specifically feminine protolanguage, communicating through the body messages that cannot be verbalized". This "feminine protolanguage" could be functionalised as a space for marking feminist reactions and resistance to patriarchal oppression.

The following section will link the historical constitution of the female mind and body as the negated complementarity of men and the resulting silencing via the depredation of feminine subjectivity to the issue of functionality in a socially constituted reality. It asks: to what functional benefit could the power dynamic of the sexes be of such robustness that the medical professional gaze on what *being women* means could percolate so seamlessly into the common sense—the everyday? Drawing on social representations of a woman's body and mind the following section stipulates a social psychodynamic inquiry.

Functional underpinnings of the *"othered"* female body— *themes, common knowledge, and identity*

The main goal of research on social representations, as Marková (2003) states, is the rehabilitation of common thinking and common knowledge, the identification, description, and analysis of the structured content and meanings of everyday knowledge conveyed in real-life situations. By introducing the notion of the topic into social representations theory, Moscovici (1993) develops an understanding of the structure and genesis within social representations and communication. Themes can be understood as prototypes of all general knowledge. Themes can be both consciously thematised in given societies and their particular contextual anchors, therefore coming to the forefront of public discourse and becoming a source of tension and conflict (Marková, 2008). In this way, themes function as "first principles", "compelling ideas", or "initial ideas" of social representations and communication (Moscovici & Vignaux, 1994/2000).

However, they may further be unconsciously mediated and implicit in our "common sense" in the form of long-lived rooted postulates of culture in attitudes, beliefs, ways of thinking, and rituals, and thus remain inaccessible to conscious explicit social thought (Marková, 2003). A subject is usually an antithetical pair, where the two components of the pair are dialectically interdependent. Marková (2003) describes the antinomic nature of human thought as underlying the generative and organising function of a theme. Through the dialectical unity of opposites, social representations are generated and transformed. Furthermore, the concept of theming explicitly focuses on the dialogic (Marková, 2003) of social representations and communication. It implies the dynamics of social knowledge, which, on the one hand, is anchored in culture and history, and, on the other hand, is maintained and reshaped through "communicative genres" (Moscovici & Marková, 2000). Social representations are a polymorphic construction, organised around themes, and their exploration refers to the uncovering of the contents of the collective historical memory (unconscious) hidden in language, whose ideas are deeply rooted and taken for granted, as well as to the social representations simultaneously domiciled in specific social and cultural contexts and negotiated in everyday life (Moscovici & Vignaux, 1994/2000).

In cultural theory, the "other" signifies those outside and implicitly subordinate to the dominant group or one's in-group. Groups lacking in power (women), identified out-groups (gay people), or "foreigners" are some examples of groups conceptually "othered". Group dynamics and othering processes lie at the heart of forging identity. Important is who we affiliate with (e.g. gender or ethnic categories) and how we compare ourselves to other groups. Gaining a positive sense of identity through comparison with negatively valued groups is common in contemporary and early Western societies alike (Said, 1978). Stallybrass and White (1986) claim that identity is constitutive via the exclusion of what and who is marked out as "low":

> ... it [the bourgeoisie] uses the whole world as its theatre in a particularly instrumental fashion, the very subjects which it politically excludes becoming exotic costumes which it assumes

in order to play out the disorders of its own identity. (...) this speaking to itself in the delirium of its repressed other has taken on considerable political significance (...) transgression, whereby bourgeois writing smashes the rigidities of its own identity by projecting itself into the forbidden territories of precisely those excluded in its own political formation, has come to seem a positive and desirable kind of romantic politics. (...) Transgression becomes a kind of reverse of counter-sublimation, undoing the discursive hierarchies and stratifications of bodies and cultures which bourgeois society has produced as the mechanism of its symbolic dominance (...) bourgeois culture constructed its self-identity by rejecting (...) the poetics of transgression reveals the disgust, fear, and desire which inform the dramatic self-representation of that culture through the "scene of its low Other". (pp. 200–202)

Joffe (2007) theorises the constitution of identity via the unconscious organisation of object representations (those people and groups relevant to our identity) according to the struggle for a sense of boundary between a pure inner space, and a polluted, outside world through anxiety-provoking situations. In this process, protection from negative feelings evoked in the self ensues by projecting unwanted material onto women's bodies at the intra-subjective level of representation but is constituted by the values and ideologies that circulate in the particular communities, cultures, and societies in which the individual is (and has even been before birth) experientially embedded within. Additionally, Joffe and Staerklé (2007) argue that identity is informed by core values within a culture. Self-control can be assumed to be one core value in Western cultures and can be understood in terms of self-control over the body, mind, and destiny (Joffe & Staerklé, 2007). As a consequence, "othering" then becomes reliant on a deficit of this valued entity, symbolising the counterpoint of what dominant groups would like to be constituted by in the West—selves in control of body, destiny, and mind.

Social groups store in the ideas they pass down through the generations not only a sense of who their disfavoured "others" are, but what aspersions are to be linked to such groups. In this very way, bifurcating sex differences and featuring each with ideas, debasements, and admirations, and eventually medical expert knowledge and practice, appears corollary. The female body and mind can be understood as generally belonging to the human category; thus, it remains attended to and under the scrutiny of social values, concurrently representing a steadfastly determined memorandum of the superiority of the male body. The service and capitalisation of this sociopolitical *trophy* varied according to its historical bearers, for example, the Christian male-coloured culture and the existence of the plague leading to the anchoring of the female body in the symbolisation of the "witch". The more society is called upon to assert being "in control", the more an *imaginable container* of all matter "out of control" finds grounds for existence. Placing the work of the evil in the silhouette of the female body, which seduces, charms, and possesses men in the name of Lucifer, allows for a solution of containment, punishment, and eventually re-establishment of control. Similarly, by placing such characteristics as feebleness, fickleness, erraticism, weak-mindedness, and capriciousness upon the female mind, similar to those of children, the social and legal subordination of women (and children) finds reasonable grounds, and tars social roles as well as rights and responsibilities. In-control men and out-of-control women.

Topical disputes within the medical field contend gender binary themes (Ferrari & Mancini, 2020) that trickle down into the everyday discourses and common sense (such as rescinding grammatical gendering in language, e.g. Magdolna et al., 2016). There is hardly any area in medicine that has seen such a striking increase in prevalence within the last decade as gender identity disorders. Psychiatric classification shifts from an understanding of gender identity disorder to gender incongruence (GI, ICD-11) or gender dysphoria (DSM-5). Furthermore, gender terminology grows increasingly varied, including non-binary gender identities being the generic term to encapsulate a spectrum of gender identities that are neither male nor female. While not recognised medical terms, the code of social law in Germany for example uses "transient, nonbinary, and intersex young persons" (Lenzen-Schulte, 2022). Further terms include bi, tri, pangender, demi-boy or demi-man, demi-girl or demi-woman, genderqueer or genderfuck. New AWMF-S3-guidelines seek to use the title "gender incongruence, gender dysphoria and trans health" to attempt to depathologise trans identity entirely, similar to the ICD-11.

It is meaningful to pursue the issue of symbolic representation in the binary thematic relation of good and evil in substantiating gender identity dynamics within this specific cultural narrative and consequentially the fracturing of these in the vortices of resistance. For example, social representations of sexual minorities are still being familiarised within a gender-binary frame of compartmentalisation (see Buetti et al., 2016; Ferrari & Mancini, 2020). Current trends seem to lead to an *I-want-to-stand-out-but-belong* attitude, which could be understood in what Bhaba (1994) names an innovative site of contestation in the act of defining the idea of society itself. By way of fracturing representations and innovating language, a modern moment oppugns the silenced battlefield of female voices that seep down from the scientific realm deep into the kernels of social think—the common sense. Ways in which this common sense are generated and organised hinge on the antinomic nature of human thinking in themata (Marková, 2003). Via the dialectical unity of opposites, social representations are generated, transformed, and thoroughly contested in our clinical practice rooms and shared attempts to give rise to communicative content, a common language, for the gendered traumas of our female patients. Just as themata are "intricately interwoven with a certain collective memory inscribed in language" (Moscovici & Vignaux, 2000, p. 182), they can show up as embedded, deep-seated, and taken-for-granted ideas in our patients' narratives.

The girl who cried pain—final comments

Medicine is but one battlefield where women must fight to be heard and believed. In a culture where women are often met with doubt and disbelief, this creates a mistrust that we often encounter in our psychotherapeutic practices as well. "When women make their own bodies an issue, it is deeply feminist" (Cleghorn, 2021, p. 23). Feminism in medicine has a long history in the fight against circumstances of "femininity" and "womanhood" entailing what American feminist author and activist Charlotte Perkins Gilman called a *denial of humanity* (Perkins Gilman, 2007). Importantly, this fight was aimed at depathologising menstruation, the allowance to live out sexual pleasure, legalising contraception, and reproductive autonomy.

One of the most recent and potent media highlights of such a feminist movement has been the #MeToo movement, which empowered women to speak out about their experiences of sexist and misogynistic abuse of power at a time when authoritarian political ideologies are on the rise around the world. Founded in 2006 by Tarana Burke via the "Me Too" Myspace page, the #MeToo movement began to help women or young girls who suffered sexual abuse, violence, harassment, or assault, and can more globally be defined as a social movement against sexual violence and sexual assault that advocates for females who survived sexual violence to speak out about their experience.

Modern movements and mentality ask for the intimately experienced and the creation and dissemination of knowledge that opposes the subliminal mystifications of male medicine and gaze. For centuries, medicine has said that a woman and her life are defined by her body and her biology. But women have never been taken seriously as reliable witnesses to the processes that are happening or have happened to their bodies. Undeniably, a knowledge that has arisen in the history of medicine is fundamental for today's understanding and practice. This chapter intended to highlight the discriminatory myths about binary gender differences and shed light on the functional underpinnings related to this social construction. From the medical theories about the diseases of women in antiquity and the first legends of hysteria to the professionalisation of gynaecology, the beginnings of public health and the development of biomedicine, medical culture, practice, and research were inseparably linked to patriarchal ideologies in a treacherous way. As Cleghorn (2021) sums up: "In the world made by men, the oppression of women was primarily legitimized by their physical and psychological constitution" (p. 30).

While the uterus was accounted for as symbolising the organ of creation and the divine purpose of woman it equally accounted for the renitent cauldron, relentlessly brewing together diseases, and thus thwarting the ideal bodily and mental state of women. Furthermore, the article argued that scrutinising such containment via narratives of rupture and re-imagination challenges the social and psychological functions, both of the one who holds power and the one over whom power is exerted, by advocating for breaking the silence and breaking old circuits of destabilising the system within which the meaning of femininity is fixed via paths of mobilising a language that separates words and meanings in prevalent social representations.

A subtle and controversial threat weaves itself through the question of breaking up old discriminatory forms of gender identities. Silenced female voices call for a time of collectively reframing questions, reassessing the data, and reinforcing each other's voices to grow audible and louder. In a world where we quarrel with increasing acceptance of the diversity of existences and forms of lives, bodies and *Lebenswelten*— people increasingly find themselves able and free to wander and search for the places and localisations where they find communities within which they feel respected and protected (as in the case example). This circumstance constitutes a *"Poli-community"* (Hannah Arendt)—not a place of identity but one of space to *Anders-sein* (trans. *"being-different"*; Schreiber, 2018, p. 13).

However, in conjunction with Adorno's claim that there cannot be a real life within a false one—that we cannot create a good space where the world around us seems to collapse—we find ourselves in a critical period of time. Struggles between an essentialist anchoring of otherness, along a dilution of rigid forms of being (e.g. the less externalised idea of home, nulling of work/office spaces in favour of home-office) and deep-felt insecurity, loneliness, and lostness in the midst of disorientation and an unbounded overture of life constructs add to possibilities of fears overtaking and defending exclusion without reason or necessity (Said, 1978). Hence our search for security is turned into its opposite. We turn inside to search for truth and home and drown in the complexity and uniqueness—we cherish and celebrate diversity while it threatens to become the fabric of our worst nightmares.

In the process of locating one's voice in the desert of silence, I would like to end on the idea of the in-between as a fruitful and disquieting space of translation where individuals, groups, and genders interact with an "other" inside a zone in which one both abandons and assumes associations (Dingwaney & Maier, 1995). The translator might exhaust all physical, emotional, and intellectual resources during the task of translation, or rather while performing "a balancing act" within the in-between. The outcome is the birth of a discourse "somewhere between sacrifice and playfulness, prison and transgression, submission to the code and aggression, obedience and rebellion, assimilation and expression—there, in this apparently empty space, its temple and its clandestinity" (Santiago, 2001, p. 38). Today's new strengthening of friend–foe thinking can be understood as a wake-up call to assert ourselves against the social pressure to conform to ever more unconditional functioning. How can we return to our own creative potential and look for other solutions in our modern lifeworld? A lifeworld that increasingly robs all of us humans of our social and feeling counterparts and subjects them to technologised optimisation expectations (Kühn, 2019). In this world, modern conditions of the feminine and masculine as sentient and felt realities of life struggle all the more with adapted definitions and the attempts to stick out and attract attention, yet not to stand out and fall out (I-want-to-stand-out-but-belong attitude).

References

American University Washington DC (2022). Overturning *Roe v. Wade*: https://american.edu/cas/news/roe-v-wade-overturned-what-it-means-whats-next.cfm

Bhabha, H. K. (1994). *The Location of Culture.* London: Routledge.

Bonomi, C. (2017). *The Cut and the Building of Psychoanalysis, Volume II: Sigmund Freud and Sándor Ferenczi.* London: Routledge.

Breuer, J., & Freud, S. (1895d). *Studies on Hysteria.* Basic Books, 1957.

Broedel, H. P. (2003). *The Malleus Maleficarum and the Construction of Witchcraft.* Manchester, UK: Manchester University Press.

Brown, I. B. (1866). *On the Curability of Certain Forms of Insanity, Epilepsy, Catalepsy, and Hysteria in Females.* London: Robert Hardwicke.

Buetti, D., Martinello, N., Moreau, N., Lapointe-Harris, T., & Ladouceur, P. (2016). Social representations of male homosexuality and their consequences for gay men: An explorative inquiry within the Canadian context. *Culture, Society & Masculinities, 8*(2): 155–173.

Cleghorn, E. (2021). *Unwell Women.* London: Weidenfeld & Nicolson.

Devereux, C. (2014). Hysteria, feminism, and gender revisited: The case of the second wave. *English Studies in Canada, 40*(1): 19–45.

Dingwaney, A., & Maier, C. (1995). *Between Languages and Cultures: Translation and Cross-Cultural Texts.* Pittsburgh, PA: University of Pittsburgh Press.

Ferrari, F., & Mancini, T. (2020). Gender binary thêmata in social representations of sexual minorities: A ten-year scoping review. *Sexuality & Culture, 24*: 2202–2229.

Freud, S. (1954). *Sigmund Freud's Letters to Wilhelm Fliess, Drafts and Notes.* M. Bonaparte, A. Freud, & E. Kries (Eds.), E. Masbacher & J. Stachey (Trans.). New York: Basic Books.

Gyimesi, J. (2019). Carlo Bonomi, "The Cut, and the Building of Psychoanalysis: Volume II. Sigmund Freud and Sándor Ferenczi". *Psychoanalysis and History, 21*(1): 123–126.

Hibbs, C. (2014). Androcentrism. In: T. Teo (Ed.), *Encyclopedia of Critical Psychology.* New York: Springer.

Joffe, H. (2007). Identity, self-control, and risk. In: G. Moloney & I. Walker (Eds.), *Social Representations and Identity.* New York: Palgrave Macmillan.

Joffe, H., & Staerklé, C. (2007). The centrality of the self-control ethos in western aspersions regarding outgroups: A social representational analysis of stereotype content. *Culture & Psychology, 13*(4): 395–418.

Jorden, E. (1603). *A Brief Discourse of a Disease Called the Suffocation of the Mother.* London.

Kors, A. C., & Peters, E. (2001). *Witchcraft in Europe 400–1700: A Documentary History.* Philadelphia, PA: University of Pennsylvania Press.

Kühn, T. (2019). Kritisch, kühn, kreativ. Der humanistische Ansatz einer analytischen Sozialpsychologie im Spiegel gesellschaftlicher Herausforderungen. In: C. Kirchhoff, T. Kühn, P. C. Langer, S. Lanwerd, & F. Schumann (Eds.), *Psychoanalytisch Denken. Sozial- und kulturwissenschaftliche Perspektiven* (pp. 35–68). Gießen, Germany: Psychosozial-Verlag.

Lenzen-Schulte, M. (2022). Transition bei Genderdysphorie: Wenn die Pubertas gestoppt wird. *Deutsches Ärzteblatt, 119*(48): A-2134 / B-17766.

Levack, B. P. (2006). *The Witch-Hunt in Early Modern Europe.* London: Pearson Education.

Magdolna, L., Lugossy, R., & Horváth, J. (2016). *UPRT 2015: Empirical Studies in English Applied Linguistics.* Csoport, Hungary: Lingua Franca.

Marková, I. (2003). *Dialogicality and Social Representations: The Dynamics of Mind.* Cambridge: Cambridge University Press.

Marková, I. (2008). The epistemological significance of the theory of social representations. *Journal for the Theory of Social Behaviour, 38*: 461–487.

Moscovici, S. (1993). *The Invention of Society: Psychological Explanations for Social Phenomena.* Cambridge: Polity.

Moscovici, S., & Marková, I. (2000). Ideas and their development: A dialogue between Serge Moscovici and Ivana Marková. In: S. Moscovici, *Social Representations.* G. Duveen (Ed.). Cambridge: Polity.

Moscovici, S., & Vignaux, G. (1994). Le concept de thêmata. In: C. Guimelli, *Structures et Transformations des Représentations Sociales* (pp. 25–72). Neuchatel, Switzerland: Delachaux et Niestlé (reprinted in Moscovici, S. (2000). *Social Representations*, G. Duveen (Ed.) (pp. 156–183). Cambridge: Polity).

Perkins Gilman, C. (2007). *The Man-Made World*. New York: Cosimo Classics.

Sadler, J. (1636). *The Sick Woman's Private Looking Glass*. London: Anne Griffin. Early English Books Online Text Creation Partnership, 2011. http://quod. lib.umich.edu/e/eebo/A11278.0001.001/1:4?rgn=div1;view=fulltext

Said, E. W. (1978). *Orientalism: Western Conceptions of the Orient*. London: Penguin.

Santiago, S. (2001). *The Space in Between: Essays on Latin American Culture*. Durham, NC: Duke University Press.

Schreiber, D. (2018). *Zu Hause. Die Suche nach dem Ort, an dem wir leben wollen* (6th edn.). Berlin: Suhrkamp Taschenbuch.

Showalter, E. (1993). Hysteria, feminism, and gender. In: S. L. Gilman, H. King, R. Porter, G. S. Rousseau, & E. Showalter (Eds.), *Hysteria Beyond Freud* (pp. 286–335). Berkeley, CA: University of California Press.

Stallybrass, P., & White, A. (1986). *The Politics and Poetics of Transgression*. Ithaca, NY: Cornell University Press.

United Nations (2012). *UN Women Data on Female Illiteracy*. https://unwomen. org/en/news/in-focus/commission-on-the-status-of-women-2012/facts-and-figures (retrieved January 25, 2023).

United Nations (2015). *The World's Women 2015: Trends and Statistics*. New York: United Nations, Department of Economic and Social Affairs, Statistics Division.

UN Women (2019). *The World for Women and Girls*. New York: United Nations Entity for Gender Equality and the Empowerment of Women.

UN Women (2023). Data on Sexual Violence Against Women and Girls. https://unwomen.org/en/what-we-do/ending-violence-against-women/facts-and-figures (retrieved January 25, 2023).

Weir Mitchell, S. (1875). Rest in nervous disease: Its use and abuse. In: E. C. Seguin (Ed.), *A Series of American Clinical Lectures* (Vol. 1, No. 4, p. 94). New York: G. P. Putnam and Sons.

Willis, T. (1681). An essay of the pathology of the brain and nervous stock. In: *Which Convulsive Diseases Are Treated of*. Samuel Pordage (Trans.). London: Printed by J. B. for T. Dring. http://name.umdl.umich.edu/A66496.0001.001

CHAPTER 6

Silencing the voices of heretics and other religions

Uta Blohm, Aleksandar Dimitrijević, and Michael B. Buchholz

It is July 27, 1656. A twenty-three-year-old man is facing what is obviously going to be the most important day of his life. Although he is already fluent in several languages, his name, Bento, makes obvious his Portuguese origin. And although he is a small-scale merchant paying off his father's debts, he is officially called before the council and the whole congregation of Amsterdam synagogue. The rabbi has prepared what is called cherem, the announcement of ostracism, extremely sharp in Bento's case, so that because of "abominable heresies that he practised and taught", no member of his community, including his siblings, will ever again be allowed to talk to him or be in any contact with him.[1]

Modest, polite, and reserved in behaviour, Bento committed only one crime: he felt passionate about asking questions and exposing logical fallacies. He wondered, for instance, about the capacity of Moses to describe his own death (by the end of the fifth Book of Moses). It was, thus, essential to silence him by isolation so that others would

---

[1] Jewish communities addressing the very questions asked by Spinoza would emerge centuries later.

not be "infected" by his questions. And when it became evident that he had spent the remaining twenty-one years of his life writing books, they would immediately be banned by both Jewish and Roman Catholic institutions, and will remain on the list of books prohibited by the Roman Catholic Inquisition (Index Librum Prohibitorum) for centuries.[2]

Few things are more natural for humans than asking questions about eternity. Our spiritual thirst, recognised in theology, philosophy, psychology, and psychoanalysis, is a universal need for each individual. Organised religions can be one of these ways, fulfilling, at the same time, many positive psychological functions for their members: hope, belonging, consolation, and encouragement. So many religions tend to insist on differences, disrupt dialogues, try to convert "infidels", and keep their believers illiterate. To silence dissonant voices, both from the outside and the inside. Think no further than the long history of prohibitions of any version of the Bible not under the control of the Roman Catholic Church, or, more specifically, Thomas More's sentencing of William Tindale, the publisher and translator of the Bible in English, to be strangled and then burned at the stake in 1536. The Bible translation into modern Greek that people without high education could read (the so-called *demotic*) was accepted by the Greek Orthodox Church only in 1997. Until then, it was only available in ancient Greek, or the very formal and outdated form of Greek (the so-called *katharevousa*) used only by the Church.

Ironically and sadly, Bento's ancestors, still bearing the family name Espinoza, were forced to leave Portugal to avoid that same destiny that ultimately befell him. After the Reconquista of 1492, the power of the Inquisition grew exponentially. Formed much earlier, the Inquisition persecuted, tortured, and murdered heretics, non-believers, Jews, converts, "witches", and scientists.

The word heresy, interestingly, comes from the ancient Greek word for choice. Heretics are, thus, those individuals who want to study or worship philosophical or religious teachings of their own choice and not as prescribed by authorities or institutions. Probably every religion encounters this, and many aim at uprooting every trace of it. Many of

---

[2] This Index itself was in use until 1966.

those who believe fervently cannot tolerate difference and even want to eradicate it.

The first book Christians banned and burnt was *Acta Pauli*, a biography of Paul of Tarsus written by an anonymous Christian but not in line with the dogma of early communities (Green & Karolides, 2005, p. 3). The largest ever collection of ancient wisdom, the Library of Alexandria, burnt not once but twice. As if the purpose was to show that all religions strive to silencing, the Library was partly destroyed by Christians around AD 400, and all the remaining manuscripts were set on fire by Muslims around 640, allegedly to heat water for public baths.

Over time, though, this practice was so widespread that it became institutionalised. In 1227, Pope Gregory IX entrusted the Inquisition to the Dominican order (Thomsett, 2010). The members of this order became known as "Domini canes"—God's hound dogs, as they did most of the interrogations, exorcisms, and executions. One of their most famous members was Girolamo Savonarola, whose preaching in the Duomo in Florence led to bonfires of vanity—burning of everything unnecessary on Piazza Della Signoria, when, allegedly, Botticelli destroyed several of his paintings—and almost ended the liberal thinking, artistic expression, and studies of ancient philosophy which define the Renaissance, only to be burned for heresy himself in 1498 (Campbell & Cole, 2017, pp. 310–313; Fletcher, 2021, p. 91).[3] Spain and Portugal expanded the Inquisition to other continents, and the ascent of Protestantism led to intensifying cruelty in the form of the Counter-Reformation, which continued until the early 1800s.[4]

Even before Bruno, Galileo, and Copernicus, excluding those who think differently seems to have been the inevitable practice in defining the credo. In the seventh century, for instance, a monk was put on trial for opposing monothelitism and exiled from Constantinople for four years, after which his tongue and right hand were cut off. Completely silenced, he died in forced exile, in today's Georgia, in 662. Less than twenty years later, he was vindicated and later came to be seen as the

---

[3] Savonarola was sentenced by Alexander VI, Borgia, possibly the most infamous of all the Popes.

[4] The emerging new Protestant churches would also come up with prejudices of their own that led to violence, and they only apologised in the twentieth century.

bearer of the true Christian faith and widely known as Maximus the Confessor.

A similar story marks the end of the life of a person whom many consider the founder of philosophy. In the year 399 BC, Socrates was sentenced to death after a one-day trial. The accusation? That he worshipped other gods and disrespected the gods of the Athenian state. He was dead the next day. At the height of the golden age of Athens, ostracism was formalised and applied legally, although, truth be told, primarily not for religious reasons.[5]

Today, nobody expects the Spanish Inquisition. But do not say that to Salman Rushdie. Although many are still subjected to similar treatments, for some people Rushdie might be the epitome of silencing as our age knows it. Yes, *The Last Temptation of Christ* by Nikos Kazantzakis was censored, and Martin Scorsese received death threats for making a movie based on it, which caused even greater havoc. Worse still with *The Life of Brian*, which remains forbidden in some countries and to members of specific communities. And, of course, the caricaturists of *Charlie Hebdo* were silenced in the cruellest possible way in a mass shooting in Paris on January 7, 2015, when twelve of them were murdered and eleven wounded. But the vicious hunt for the Indian-born novelist lasted almost thirty-five years, most of which he had to spend in isolation. Finally, Rushdie was attacked on stage on August 12, 2022, and repeatedly stabbed in the face, neck, and abdomen. His life was saved only after a lengthy medical procedure, but not his right eye and ability to use one hand. The reason? In 1988, Rushdie published a novel, *The Satanic Verses*, in which he mentioned one of the holy books and one of the alleged prophets. Artistic imagination was enough for Iran's then religious and ideological dictator to officially curse Rushdie, despite not having read the book himself, and offer a two million dollar reward to his murderer, after which a host of fanatics opened the hunt. The author, already holding double UK–US citizenship, had to hide and was under constant surveillance and protection. After repeated assassination

---

[5] Ostrakon means a piece of broken pottery, which became a voting instrument, given that as many as 6,000 people had to vote against someone for that person to be exiled, and shards of pottery were everywhere.

attempts, some of which included bombings, the only mystery is how the assassins do not see Rushdie's survival as a miracle and his life as martyrdom.[6]

On a more general level, the aforementioned monothelitic and monophysitic controversies[7] are, simultaneously, illustrations for another, and quite fundamental, form of religious silencing: the silencing of any emotions and wishes related to the body. Centuries-long discussions about whether Jesus Christ had one (divine) or two (both divine and human) wills and natures—and if two, how they disentangled from one another—showed a struggle with an overemphasis on the transcendental, supernatural, and superhuman. While for the ancients, the divine was (in) nature, physis, beginning with Plato's expression "beyond nature" in his description of the world of ideas, in his *Republic*, the slow change of focus led to the anthropology of Socrates, to Christian ethics and instructions for everyday life. The demand that every Christian should "be perfect as your heavenly father is perfect" (Matthew, 5:48) inspired the medieval ideal of *imitatio Christi*. Because the gospels do not mention that Jesus had a family, particularly devout Christians opted for living in deserts and caves or on small, elevated platforms, and to live, as all the Catholic priests still do, in total celibacy and avoidance of any bodily pleasures. The seventh-century monk from Mount Sinai, John, known as "of the Ladder", or in Greek "Climacus", wrote one of the most famous instructions for this kind of life. His nickname, which even Kierkegaard used as a pseudonym, refers to his only surviving manuscript, *The Ladder of Divine Ascent*, a manual for the overcoming of one's body and individual soul and bringing them closer to God. There are thirty of these ladders described, the first one being the renunciation of life, followed by advice related to overcoming sins and achieving virtues.

---

[6] Muslims are in today's world perpetrators of religious violence (and victims themselves) as well as victims of political persecution, for example, in China. The situation is increasingly complex.

[7] This refers to centuries-long debates about the number of wills and persons Jesus was believed to have (divine and/or human), as well as possible boundaries and relations between them.

The example of chronologically perhaps the first among the Christian ascetics, Anthony of Egypt, also known as "Anthony of the Desert" and "the Hermit", initiated the fasting of Advent and Lent imposed on all, which twice a year lasts six weeks. Another technique of the so-called mortification of the body, loosely connected to the vague statement "I chastise my body" (1 Corinthians, 9:27), was self-flagellation, which also existed in other religious traditions. Because Jesus was poor, some Christians renounced all possessions and comforts, including beds and mattresses or heating. The attempt to overcome everything connected or stemming from the body included renouncing our most fundamental needs, like foregoing sleep for prolonged periods, and communication with others, practised by the monks of diverse traditions who take the vows of silence that may last for years.

Relying on the "supernatural overcoming of the natural", to use a phrase from John Climacus again, monks, priests, and believers have for centuries been silencing their desires, emotions, and needs, all too often, although not always, going into the extremes of avoiding any pleasure, insisting on absolute chastity, living without any social contacts. If nothing else, due to the fear of an omnipotent and unknowable god or punishment in the mysterious afterlife, millions have silenced every voice they were told they had to silence. Along the way, this has created misery and frustration in the lives of countless persons, widely present practices of hypocritical gratification, and whole societies estranged from pleasure, exchange, and authenticity.

Christian silencing of its Jewish roots and attempts at establishing a dialogue

In the first part of this chapter, we have illustrated the silencing that institutions of various religions perform against their members. These individual cases are now well documented and partly even romanticised. But unfortunately, religious groups tend to silence whole other religious groups, even to the level of genocide. Conversions have been enforced in all parts of the world, and religious wars have devastated Europe for centuries and made Arabs, Ottomans, and Europeans bring devastation to other continents. One might even wonder whether religions have to act like that because it is difficult for them to negotiate, given that they all rely on the authority of all-powerful and all-knowing god(s). At the same time, it seems that the silenced religions find ways to infiltrate into the prevailing ones so that we can see traces of Judaism in Christianity, both of them in Islam, native religions in Latin American Catholicism, and Slavic religions in Orthodox Christianity.[8]

Of all the histories of religious silencing, none is more tragic than the Christian silencing of Judaism,[9] because if the history of Christian denial did not lead to the Shoah it definitely contributed.[10]

Jewish communities were persecuted throughout European Christian history. This happened in particular during the crusades and the afore-mentioned Reconquista to regain Spain from the Arabs. The Talmud was forbidden and burnt throughout Europe, on papal orders, countless times after the twelfth century (for a detailed list, see Green & Karolides, 2005, pp. 109ff.). In the early twentieth century, Jewish communities in Russia faced pogroms, and between 1933 and 1945 an attempt was made to murder all European Jews led by Nazi Germany and supported to various degrees by some other European governments (while facing meagre resistance). But how did it all start? What was the path that led to this?

Anti-Jewish prejudice comes in many forms. One of the foundations that make it possible is silencing the rich connections and mutual influences between Judaism and Christianity. The underlying belief of Christian anti-Jewish[11] teachings is one of Christian superiority. A new group had replaced the old group of believers and made it irrelevant.

---

[8] A perfect example in this respect is the *Mnemosyne Atlas* by Aby Warburg, which showed how Renaissance Florentine paintings of biblical scenes were under the heavy influence of the then-contemporary Arabic books, which were in turn heavily influenced by ancient Greek manuscripts. In a Christian context, this process is called inculturation.

[9] This is not to say that Jewish prejudice against Christians does not exist. Given these historical circumstances, it often takes a long time to meet on equal footing. For very good reasons, Jewish participants in dialogue may be wary if they can trust the Christian side or if an attempt at proselytising may come their way.

[10] Shoah is used instead of the more familiar term, the Holocaust, which is problematic because it can mean sacrifice.

[11] It is debated whether it is more appropriate to use the term anti-Jewish or anti-Semitic. The term anti-Jewish was commonly used for Christian prejudice since it was assumed that it did not include a racial/ethnic component such as the anti-Semitism of National Socialism.

This Christian belief is already portrayed in the structure of the two parts of the Christian Bible. The first part consists of the Hebrew scriptures and is traditionally called the Old Testament. The second part was written in the first century CE in Greek and contains uniquely Christian books, mainly four books (gospels), which describe the story about the life of Jesus Christ ("Christ" being Greek for "Messiah"), and the letters (which are older than the gospels) to communities outside Jerusalem. This part of the Christian Bible is called the New Testament in the official versions. In an attempt to place equal value on the first part, suggestions have been made to use the terms First and Second Testament (Zenger, 1993), and sometimes in Christian communities, the term "Hebrew Bible" is used. The Hebrew Bible is not identical to the Jewish Bible since the biblical books are ordered differently in the Hebrew Bible and Christian Old Testaments. What is most important for our topic is that the so-called Old Testament orders these books in the Christian hermeneutic framework as having their culmination in the story of Jesus as portrayed in the New Testament.

There are many individual points of silencing related to the central theological tenets. For example, the words in Mark 12:31: "Love thy neighbour as thyself" are often considered Christian, whereas they have their roots in the Hebrew parts of the Christian Bible (Leviticus 19:18). Jesus was quoting Hebrew scriptures, not introducing an entirely new and radical teaching. More widely known perhaps (and still widely used in common culture) is the stereotype of the Old Testament God as the one of wrath and the New Testament God as the one of love.[12]

The seeds of Christian bias were sown in the New Testament, even though, strictly speaking, the Christian communities had not yet formed entities separate from the Jewish ones at the time of its writing. It was probably essential for these emerging communities to over-emphasise every point difference and underline their originality. So, in John's gospel, the Jews appear as the enemy of Jesus, and Paul discusses in his most famous letter to the flourishing Christian community in Rome the relationship between the Christian community and "Israel" (the allegedly chosen people). The other three gospels in

---

[12] This is a strange irony since Jews have been oppressed and persecuted by Christians throughout history and have every right to say, "That's what Christian love means."

the New Testament are more closely related, and here the enemies of Jesus are the Pharisees. In European Christian consciousness, the word Pharisee can stand for rabbi or Jew. When a Jewish scholar in the nineteenth century suggested that Jesus may have been a Pharisee, he caused outrage (Heschel, 1998).[13]

Christianity, as is well known, did not start as a European religion but became the main religion in Europe through its involvement with the Roman Empire, where Jewish communities formed minority groups. Christianity or the churches started as one among many groups within ancient Israel. This was a messianic group which believed that its messiah was crucified by the occupying power (the Romans) in conjunction with the local elite, who saw this popular man as a threat to their power. Communities of believers in Jesus Christ grew and consisted of people who were originally Jewish and those who were not. Within the Christian community, the question arose to what degree non-Jewish members were bound by Jewish practices (and law), particularly those related to food and circumcision.[14]

Nevertheless, from the perspective of the Roman Empire, the early Christian communities were falsely considered Jewish. It was not unusual for Jewish communities to have Godfearers in their midst: people

---

[13] In Germany, there is a type of coffee with alcohol called "pharisee" to symbolise that it is as untrustworthy as Jews are considered to be. It is still on the menu, even in Berlin.

[14] Jan Assmann (1999) named this a "normative inversion"—if one religion demands liquids to be drunk in the morning, after conversion, the true believer is demanded to eat food. First, stand while praying, and the others lay down on the floor. Just do the opposite to achieve a maximum difference—and this demonstrates that one's past can/ must be silenced for the new "true believer". When you pray, hold your hand's fingers up while leaning palms against each other; after conversion, pray with folded hands and observe that the fingers of the right hand are above those of the left (or inverse). Until the nineteenth century in Europe, people—Calvinists, Catholics, Lutherans, and others—had to document that they knew the "correct" manner. Otherwise, in the many religious wars, they were threatened by death. "By their signs, you will recognize them"—these were the words of Jesus (Matthew 7:16), based on a long tradition in Asia Minor where they had not only one but up to 150 gods. One had to document where one belonged. These practices of correct gestures and correct praying words could be exchanged when, with a conversion, people changed their groups. Only the Jewish practice of circumcision could not be reversed.

who were part of the community but did not convert precisely because circumcision was problematic from a Greek or Roman perspective but faith in one God was attractive (when one had abandoned the Greek/Roman pantheon). It can be argued that messianic communities took over because they allowed full membership without circumcision (Sybil Sheridan in a seminar at Leo Baeck College, London, in 2001). At some point, some of these messianic communities consisted entirely of non-Jewish members. It is debated at what point the two communities formed separate entities.

The very fact that the writings of the church fathers contain anti-Jewish polemics and warn against attending services in synagogues—because, among other things, "Jewish" equalled "satanic" if one follows John's gospel. This is a testimony such that people were confused about their allegiances—which must have forced them to tell many lies or to keep themselves silent.

A profound theological problem arose: if Jewish equalled satanic, what consequences did that have for the belief that Jesus was of Jewish origin, given that his mother was Jewish, as well as the whole community in which he grew up? Unfortunately, many Christians would not know this, as the New Testament stories which make this obvious, for example, the one that describes Jesus's circumcision, may be silenced via the omission from the list of readings for church Sunday services.[15]

Another more serious example is that Jews have been held responsible for the death of Jesus and, as such, have been accused of deicide. Good Friday, the day when Christians traditionally read the stories of the crucifixion of Jesus, could be a dangerous day for Jewish populations in Europe.

Anti-Jewish bias can also be found in academic Christian studies, even though these claim to be neutral or scientific. To give one example: a New Testament scholar, Joachim Jeremias, considered Jesus the radical person who introduced the word "Abba" (father) for God as a form of solid criticism of Judaism. It took a PhD to study Jewish sources and

---

[15] This is also related to the dogma of the immaculate conception, which granted Jesus the divine origin, nature, and will. Church councils were then focused on the differentiation between the divine and human in him, but not on his Jewish origin.

discover that there is nothing new about Jesus using the word father for God (Böckler, 1999).

Also, Judaism at the time of the New Testament and rabbinic Judaism were called Late Judaism by Christiam scholars as if Judaism had ceased to exist as a living entity after the rise of Christianity.

The same anti-Jewish bias can be found in Christian art too. Throughout history, Jews have been portrayed in Christian churches with a blindfold because they do not accept Jesus as their Messiah. Another critical point is that for centuries all the biblical characters were represented with typical European facial features, clothes, and objects. Even the most extraordinary paintings contain this bias as a rule: when Holbein the father portrayed the circumcision of baby Jesus (now in the Alte Pinakothek in Munich), the scene is taking place in medieval Europe; all of Raphael's or Leonardo's Madonnas (a possible pinnacle of Christian art) are pretty Italian women in Florentine garments; even when Michelangelo painted the ceiling of the Sistine chapel with exclusively Old Testament motifs, his sabotage (or an act of revenge to Pope Julius II) went unnoticed because visually there was nothing Jewish in the frescoes. So generalised was this silencing that the first painting in which Jesus is dressed as a Jewish man was Marc Chagall's *White Crucifixion* from 1938 (now in the Art Institute of Chicago).[16]

It is mind-blowing to think that the so-called German Christians in Nazi Germany tried to create some Aryan interpretation of the New Testament by portraying Jesus as a positive figure in a dark Jewish world. In the aftermath of the Shoah, something strange and new happened: Jews and Christians started talking to each other. There were, of course, earlier attempts at developing a dialogue: from the Convivencia in the Arab Andalucía, especially in the twelfth century,

---

[16] Although that is not an example of religious art, there had been no traces of Jewish music in symphonic and operatic traditions until the end of the nineteenth century. For instance, the famous "Coro Hebraico" is pure Verdi and is now Italy's unofficial second national anthem. The first time we hear an unmistakable klezmer tune in a symphony is in Gustav Mahler's First Symphony, at the beginning of the third movement, right after the double-basses have played "Frère Jacques" in the tempo of a funeral march. Mahler had to mark the movement *attacca*, so there would be no break after it and no time for otherwise very loud protests. Still, he was fired from the Budapest Opera roughly one year after the symphony premiered in late 1889.

to the efforts by Albertus Magnus and Meister Eckart around that same time, to Martin Luther, who for the translation of the Bible had learned his Hebrew from rabbis, and Nicolas Cusanus bringing Christians, Jews, and Muslims together in the sixteenth century.

Sometimes the very place of these contemporary encounters was Germany, where the twentieth-century genocide originated. The Shoah happened in Christian Europe, and many of the perpetrators were Christians, or, at least, many Nazi perpetrators had been baptised. So, the question arose: how had Christian culture contributed to the attempt to kill all European Jews and destroy/annihilate Jewish culture and history (or convert Jewish history for the only purpose of displaying it in museums)?

Jewish-Christian dialogue in the twentieth century has sometimes been described as "tables being turned". Whereas in the past, Christians felt they were the ones in possession of truth and silenced Jews through attempts of conversion or violence and murder, some Christians[17] now started listening and often found that they had very little to say. Some Christian churches now state explicitly that Jews are the chosen people no less than Christians (for example, in 1980, one Protestant Church in Germany changed its constitution—"Rheinischer Synodalbeschluss"). This is progress—however, it is a problem when Jews are being defined from the outside (Jonathan Magonet, personal communication, July 2009). Various attempts have been made to describe Jewish–Christian relations as sibling relations (Judaism being the older brother) or Judaism being the parent religion. Still, it may perhaps be best to describe Jewish–Christian relations as an open wound (Ritschl, 1986).[18]

All this opened a process of painful soul-searching for some Christians involved in the dialogue and a review of the Christian tradition as it has evolved over the last two millennia. A body of research was created into Christian anti-Jewish or anti-Semitic teachings and their origins. The nature of dialogue began to change or sometimes changes

---

[17] Some others, including the then reigning pope, in the 1940s and after that, helped Nazi perpetrators to flee to Argentina.

[18] Unfortunately, groups such as "Jews for Jesus", which aim at converting Jews, still exist. They often target vulnerable people with mental health issues, who are not uncommon among religious zealots.

when people meet with sincerity and listen to each other. People no longer meet as victims and accused but as humans with complicated histories. If and when that happens, it is sometimes possible to talk openly about one's religious tradition and identity and how to relate to these stories in the light of history and modern science.

The next section delivers a psychoanalytic case history, documenting the forces of silencing, which could be invalidated during treatment.

Seeing lies—a modality of hearing silencing

Paul was an artist in his early thirties and worked in an institution where his sense for aesthetics, poetry, and design was highly esteemed. Moreover, he was in love with a young woman he wanted to marry. "She is the woman I want to marry," he informed his therapist.

However, sometimes he was so depressed that he thought of committing suicide, and he did not have even a hunch of an idea why. So, he looked for consolation, and when he snuggled up with his girlfriend, he became quiet inside.

We began a psychoanalytic treatment and were meeting three times per week. His history was centred upon the Christian faith in extreme Catholic rigour. Praying rituals before and after eating, attending services, praying in the evening, speaking softly, and specific ways to dress—so embarrassing in school!

In one session, he returned to the conditions he needed to fall asleep. He confessed that he needed to touch his girlfriend's bosom, and only then could he fall asleep. I wondered about this detail and asked him to tell me more about that. He was the fourth child born to his mother, and one year after his birth, a brother followed. He had never thought he might have had his mother's warm bosom. "This is so obvious," he said, wondering why he had never thought about this. That was the first time he cried in sessions. Deeply dejected, he returned to the next session with a question, "If that's the reason, how can I get rid of my depression?" We talked about the role of siblings and the feelings of envy he felt when he went into the room and saw his mother with his younger brother at her bosom—how angry that made him! How sad! Already at that early time in life! Was this the origin of his depression? Then an outbreak of rage: how could his mother dare to have so many children? How could his parents, such devout Christians, produce one child after another? Another year after his younger brother, a sister followed. He was full of rage against his father—without responsibility for the family, child after child! Then, one day coming home from school, he discovered that his pious father had an extramarital affair!

It took us several sessions before he understood that his severe depression was based on losing his mother's warmth and closeness too early and that he, as a grown-up person, could work on breaking away from this backwards-looking desire.

One of his older siblings had given birth to a girl when he was twelve. When she was five, he had a lovely and funny relationship with her. They jumped around and played games with each other. He, now seventeen years old, let her sit on his lap and read to her, and sometimes he stayed at her bedside until she fell asleep in the evening. However, one day she uttered: "I wish you were dead!" He was slightly shocked, as he did not understand why she said this. Just for fun?

When he returned to this memory a second or third time, I told him that his niece might have said something he would never dare. To wish someone dead! Incredible! In such a religious family! He remembered how intense his hatred against his father was, and he confessed, interrupted by tears, that he recently thought that his father, growing older and suffering from forgetfulness, might finally die after all. He confessed these thoughts in a mixture of guilt plus expectation of being punished—that I delivered an interpretation, showing how bad he is and how infantile. I drew his attention to this double category of what he expected and said I was wondering—why punishment? For what? He asked if I believed such thoughts were not a sin. I responded believing that I should also believe that such thoughts would have power, but they are only thoughts! However, I could imagine how firm his conviction must have been in the religious family world he grew up in. Here, evil thoughts come from a bad soul, so dark and sinister that such a soul could never expect to ascend to heaven for eternal salvation.

Next session, he came and opened the session with nervous laughter. Back home after the last session, alone in his kitchen, he dared to whisper to himself, "Dad, I want you to die!" Very calm, then louder and then really loud! And nothing happened! He laughed so loud about this discovery! He pondered if his niece might have done a similar experiment—what happens if I dare speak out "silenced thoughts"? It took us a sequence of sessions until he felt his silenced conviction: having, or even worse, speaking out silenced thoughts, being condemned to hell! Once, he remembered how an elder brother had raised his finger and warned him that he never! never! never! dare to speak out such thoughts. He was silenced and made to believe such thoughts might become true. He had believed that thoughts have such strong effects. How was he convinced that evil thoughts could come true?

In one session, I added that psychoanalysis had named this "belief in the omnipotence of thought", and I told him as an illustration that children sometimes steal sweets, and when the adult person asks them whether they know where the chocolate is, they respond: "No!" And then, children are so surprised that adults do *not* know what is happening.[19] They cannot read the child's thoughts! To realise what was going on in his family beyond pious practices, and that others did not know what was happening—his mother with an unfaithful husband, his niece testing him, and he with an enormous rage against his brother and his father! He had defended against this knowledge by regression in behaving like a baby when the time to sleep came—this was the real shock! Like a baby who did not know. Or better, a child whose thoughts were self-silenced because he had believed that thoughts would become true! That he would have the power to kill. The utterance of his little niece must have been an attempt to find out if her thoughts could kill him!

The patient suffered from being forced to convert—not to speak his thoughts, as thoughts were maintained to be dangerous, influential acts harming others. This conviction produces a logical knot not only in children but in adults, too. You are taught that some of your thoughts can harm you; therefore, you are *instructed* not to think specific thoughts. However, the ban or prohibition does not aim at specific thoughts but at the ability to think in general. Once you try not to think specific thoughts, you quickly realise that you are thinking the

---

[19] This is taken from a narrative delivered by the founder of conversation analysis, Harvey Sacks (Sacks & Jefferson, 1992, p. 114). Sacks reported his reading of a supervision Victor Tausk had received from Sigmund Freud. The headline "seeing lies" is also taken from Sacks.

forbidden thought. The religious lesson achieves the opposite effect! The recipient of the interdiction, willing to follow the instruction, cannot escape this logical trap. The effect is considerable intimidation, which children turn to when they try to comply. They become shy.

They experience a kind of conversion which strongly parallels the history of religion. Religious teachers cannot use followers who are entirely inhibited in thinking. So, many distinctions were historically introduced to "heal" the effect of over-intimidation. The most important one is that of "good" and "bad"—there are "good thoughts" (e.g. in prayers) and "bad thoughts", and there is another distinction between "doing" and "thinking". The recipient of such instructions can "show" how good intentions and thoughts are in him or her—to *show* this publicly is the meaning of "to behave"; the distinction between visible behaviour and invisible thoughts is established.

The distinction between "good" and "bad" thoughts is the moralistic founding act of the superego and its installation in a child's mind. Without such a distinction, many religions would not have survived. Without such a discovery, a child could never move a single step, and she falls silent. The discovery that others do not know what is going on makes one free to think of one's thoughts and to communicate selected thoughts, which contributes to the process of individualization. However, there might be circumstances that make this discovery traumatic, and intimidation and shyness are installed in a child's mind. A child is being silenced.

Conclusion

Silencing seems to be present in various religious institutions and on their different layers. We presented multiple examples of silencing disobedient individuals or entire religious groups, and one clinical illustration of the consequences of this process. Our examples were arbitrarily chosen, and other authors could have come up with different ones. There is no doubt that religious groups and institutions need to work a lot on overcoming the tendency towards silencing, but the ongoing interreligious dialogue gives hope that the situation is not entirely dark, as religion can be a force for both good and evil. We hope that our small contribution will lead to further studies about how silencing can and has been overcome.

References

Assmann, J. (1999). Conversion, piety and loyalism in Ancient Egypt. In: J. Assmann & G. G. Ṣṭrumzah (Eds.), *Studies in the History of Religions: Vol. 83. Transformations of the Inner Self in Ancient Religions*. Leiden, the Netherlands: Brill.

Böckler, A. (1999). *Gott als Vater im Alten Testament. Traditionsgeschichtliche Untersuchungen zur Entstehung und Entwicklung eines Gottesbildes.* Wuppertal, Germany: Kaiser Gütersloher Verlagshaus.

Campbell, S. J., & Cole, M. W. (2017). *A New History of Italian Renaissance Art.* London: Thames & Hudson.

Fletcher, S. (2021). *Religion.* In: G. Campbell (Ed.), *The Oxford Illustrated History of the Renaissance.* Oxford: Oxford University Press.

Green, J., & Karolides, N. J. (2005). *Encyclopedia of Censorship.* New York: Infobase.

Heschel, S. (1998). *Abraham Geiger and the Jewish Jesus.* Chicago, IL: University of Chicago Press.

Ritschl, D. (1986). *The Logic of Theology.* London: SCM.

Sacks, H., & Jefferson, G. (1992). *Lectures on Conversation.* G. Jefferson (Ed.). Introduction by Emanuel A. Schegloff. Oxford: Basil Blackwell, 1995.

Thomsett, M. C. (2010). *The Inquisition: A History.* Jefferson, NC: McFarland.

Zenger, E. (1993). *Das Erste Testament. Die jüdische Bibel und die Christen* (3rd edn.). Düsseldorf, Germany: Patmos.

CHAPTER 7

Silence in the classroom: suppressing (gifted) students' curiosity and creativity

Ana Altaras Dimitrijević

From private study rooms to public reading halls, places of intellectual activity are often associated with sustained and pervasive silence. In light of this, requiring students to be quiet during class appears as a reasonable intervention to establish the proper setting for them to pick up, process, and reflect on the contents taught. However, effective learning at school thrives not just on silence; clearly, there must also be opportunities for students to speak up in class—to utter surprise or bewilderment, raise a question, express excitement about a topic, and/or signal their progress to the teacher. Unfortunately, evidence shows that schools tend to suppress not only those utterances and behaviours which may disrupt the learning process, but also those that communicate a student's intense curiosity or creative insights about a subject. The focus of this chapter is precisely on acts of silencing which occur when particular students, that is, those who by most standards would be labelled gifted, voice more inquisitiveness and eagerness to learn than their teachers, peers, or the education system as a whole are willing to support. The chapter's first aim is to document this phenomenon and its various instances, by drawing on findings and cases reported in the literature, as well as on examples from the author's own work with gifted students. As a second goal, the chapter seeks to weigh the gravity of this phenomenon—and the residues it leaves in the lives and minds of affected students—while also addressing the beliefs and circumstances that have sustained the disquieting practice of silencing giftedness well into the twenty-first century.

Instances of silencing giftedness at school

Psychological accounts of giftedness have come a long way from the nineteenth-century notion that true genius cannot be silenced and "if hindered and thwarted, will fret and strive until the hindrance is overcome" (Galton, 1869, p. 38). Admittedly, gifted children are still characterized as having a "rage to master" (Winner, 1996)—that is, an intense drive to acquire the knowledge and skills of the domain in which they display high ability; nevertheless, contemporary views on giftedness also recognise that this intrinsic motivation can easily be undermined by inadequate child-rearing and educational practices. The assumption that the gifted will make themselves heard in any circumstances has thus been largely replaced in favour of the empirically more tenable view that giftedness will actualise itself only with proper environmental support, with schools playing a non-negligible part in this process (see e.g. Baccassino & Pinnelli, 2023; Sternberg & Davidson, 2005). Not infrequently, however, the role executed by schools is that of suppressing rather than nurturing high ability and the drive to learn. The silencing of gifted students at school takes many forms and occurs at many levels, as will be outlined in the sections that follow.

Silenced by the crowd (or self-silencing to please the crowd)

For many gifted children in the Western world, coming from small nuclear families into a school community of peers may be the first moment to realise that they have little or nothing in common with other students (Gross, 2004) when it comes to their academic interests and skills (which, after all, are at the center of attention in schools). And while interpersonal maladjustment and low social competence are not inherent to high ability (see e.g. Lee et al., 2012), this awareness of being different from their peers can make gifted students feel acutely uncomfortable and threaten their social relationships (Gross, 1999). As postulated by the "stigma of giftedness paradigm" (e.g. Coleman & Cross, 2000; Cross et al., 1995), gifted students (a) desire normal social interactions; (b) learn that others will treat them differently when aware of their giftedness; and (c) employ various strategies to manage information about themselves and thus attain the desired social outcomes. What this means is that, often, they will "act swiftly to conform to the social or behavioral norms of their age-group" (Gross, 1999, p. 211) and conceal or even deny their abilities to gain peer acceptance. As a striking example, Gross (1998, 1999, 2004) reports that within four weeks of entering school the majority of the precocious children in her study regressed in their reading performance—beginning to "mumble and stumble over words" which they could fluently read at home—or even stopped reading altogether, pretending to be analphabets (pp. 176–177). This manoeuvre of muting their skills to be more like their classmates is used by gifted children throughout school, so that ultimately, "several cannot recall a time [...] when this has not been an automatic survival mechanism, accepted as a painful but necessary part of living" (Gross 2004, p. 272). Other research also indicates that, in the course of their schooling, students become increasingly less willing to openly show or speak about their performance and skills, for fear of damaging their peer status (Händel et al., 2013).

A legitimate question, of course, is whether the above behaviours are indeed an instance of being silenced or rather a form of self-silencing that takes place in anticipation of a peer rejection which might only be imagined. Unfortunately, research has repeatedly shown that being "brilliant and studious" is not a popular combination (Cramond & Martin, 1987) and that gifted students do face "anti-achievement peer pressure" (Moon, 2009), including overt negative reactions to their intellectual pursuits and active attempts to silence them. An early study by Torrance (1963, in Benbow & Stanley, 1996) found, for instance, that highly creative sixth-graders suffered "open aggression and hostility, criticism, rejection and indifference" from their less creative peers, even when they were all engaged in a cooperative activity, the successful completion of which would mean a reward for the whole group. The importance of not being earnest is also evidenced by the experiences of the students studied by Gross (1998), such as Emma, a gifted teenager who attempted to share her interest in a current political issue with her schoolmates, only to be ostentatiously shunned by them until she resumed the usual conversation on clothes and make-up. In some cases, the silencing of gifted students can even take the form of blatant violence, as in the case of "African American urban teenagers who try to achieve [...] in a hostile environment created by groups or gangs who terrorize [them] [and] intimidate them with death threats" (Benbow & Stanley, 1996, p. 259). According to a more recent study (Händel et al., 2013), high achievement in certain subjects still tends to trigger negative peer reactions, explaining why gifted students rather refrain from talking about their intellectual pursuits.

Silenced by the system

One might argue that the examples described above are all cases of gifted students being "silenced by the crowd", not by the school as such. In other words, the school would just happen to be the place, but not an agent of silencing the gifted. A contrary viewpoint, and one that appears closer to the truth, is that the concept and structure of compulsory education are such that the school very much contributes to suppressing individual gifts and talents. Thus, it would not (just) be the peer group at school, but the school itself that pressures gifted students to fit in—socially, as well as intellectually.

What is it about schools that turns them into temples of silencing? As revealed in Inbar's (1996) metaphor study, it is not uncommon for educators to perceive students "as receptacles that have to be filled, as clay that has to be moulded or as helpless buds that have to be nourished" (p. 91). According to the author, such images invite the use of authoritative control and imply that students ought to quietly receive the instruction provided, since, obviously, "Receptacles, clay, pots and flowers cannot complain" (Inbar, 1996, p. 84). The same type of muteness or lack of an individual voice is conveyed by a school-related metaphor from the popular culture—that of "another brick in the wall"—coined to illustrate how schools tend to control and subjugate children instead of educating them (Roger Waters, cited in Myers, 2015). In line with this, the metaphors produced by the students in Inbar's (1996) study often entailed images of being "caged", "trapped", "captive", or "imprisoned" in school. Together with the educators' responses, these metaphors clearly reveal "the inherent tensions and contradictions" of compulsory education: on the one side, it aims at the fulfilment of each individual's intellectual and creative potential (see e.g. *Law on the fundamentals of the education system* of the Republic of Serbia); on the other, it follows a one-size-fits-all approach that largely disregards individual differences. As concluded by Inbar: "Education, even if it takes place in groups, is an individualized process. Schooling, on the other hand, is a group solution to education. It is based on compliance, on standards and averages [...]" (pp. 90–91).

The fact that schooling is based on "standards and averages" hardly benefits any student but has particularly adverse consequences for those who deviate most from the average—unless, of course, they are provided special educational attention. In the words of an eleventh-grader from Inbar's study, the school is like a "garden with different flowers, some of them are well cared for and flourishing, others are falling and withering; [...] the weeds should be plucked" (Inbar, 1996, p. 89). Counterintuitive as it may sound, the "withering flowers" and "weeds" often turn out to be gifted students, as schools offer relatively few special provisions for the development of their abilities, that is, they often fail to make the necessary adjustments in terms of content, pacing, and/or grouping that would be expected in an inclusive classroom. It is precisely this state of affairs that has led scholars in the field to conclude that gifted students are neglected by the system (Benbow & Stanley, 1996) and are "at risk in a place called school" (Feldhusen & Hoover, 1984), or that being highly creative is not an asset but a handicap in most classrooms (Gowan et al., 1979, in Kim, 2008). Even when it comes to universities, it has long been noted that "most of our institutions of higher learning offer intellectual fare distressingly below the digestive capacity of the gifted. [...] Usually such a student does well, and the teacher rejoices, but in many cases the teacher should feel less joy than guilt, for he has, intentionally, beckoned the gifted student downward toward mediocrity rather than upward toward maximum self-development" (Allport, 1960, cited in Benbow & Stanley, 1996, p. 252).

Again, one might argue, in defence of the education system, that not actively providing for gifted students is not tantamount to silencing them. Surely, if these students came up to the teacher and asked for more input and challenge, their request would not be ignored or denied. "Ask and you shall receive", right?

"Please, Sir, I want some more" … explicit silencing by the teacher

Yet, the experiences of gifted students who did ask their teachers for more tell a more complex story. Surely, and fortunately, one could give countless examples of educators who will happily provide the extra materials and challenge that these students require. At the same time, there is also plenty of evidence to the contrary—to acts of silencing that go beyond overlooking the gifted students in the classroom to directly denying the fulfilment of their needs, even when these are expressed quite clearly and explicitly. The cases of such silencing described below stem from my own work with gifted students and their parents (unless otherwise indicated by the reference) and have all taken place within the last ten years, in metropolitan settings, within the German (see the case of David below) or Serbian (see the cases of Vincent and Nick) educational system.

Cut down on the questions

The most straightforward and probably most common form of silencing gifted students is by curtailing their questions and asking/telling them to quit a topic of interest. Of note, while indeed claiming the teacher's attention and involvement, the utterances that are thus being silenced are generally not made in a way that interrupts the teacher or other students in the class. Nevertheless, instead of taking the time to respond to the question or refer the student to relevant sources of information, the teacher will typically stop to explain that this is neither the time nor the place for questions. In some cases, the teacher may even go so far as to openly accuse the student of asking or, indeed, of "being too much" and "always having to have a question" (citations of two gifted students).

This is precisely the scenario experienced by Vincent, a gifted second grader, whose immense intellectual curiosity was particularly drawn to chemistry. In his first year of schooling, Vincent had already learned to bridle this curiosity and focus on the task at hand, so that by second grade he was finishing his schoolwork ahead of time and consistently earning the highest grades. It was his mother's expectation that he would be praised for these efforts in self-regulation and allowed to learn something new and challenging in the spare time gained through his swiftness. The feedback she received at school, however, was rather indicative of the teacher's efforts to fully muzzle Vincent's inquisitiveness: specifically, the teacher informed the mother that things were "somewhat better now than before; before, it was just impossible to live with all this talk about chemistry". The teacher also attributed this "improvement" to an eye-to-eye talk with Vincent, in which she (the teacher) had told him to "come to his senses, realise that he is not in high school but in second grade, and forget about chemistry". Fortunately, Vincent's mother did not let herself be silenced, but went on to consult the school principal, who eventually allowed Vincent to be pulled out of class every once in a while, to have individual lessons with the chemistry teacher working at the same school.

Erase and don't show what you know

Going a step further from asking gifted students to give up on what they want to know, is telling them to forget and disregard what they already know. A striking example to illustrate this kind of silencing is that of David—a mathematically precocious boy, who entered school with a fully formed understanding of positive and negative numbers (apart from being able to read and write). At the beginning of second grade, David's class was given a simple test to screen the level of attained addition and subtraction skills with numbers up to 20; the test also featured the following "odd" question: $2 - 6 = ?$ Given his mathematical skills, David wrote -4 as his response. This, however, was graded as a mistake and resulted in a one-point deduction on the test, with no word of explanation or expression of interest from the teacher. Highly upset and confused, David confronted the teacher with what he thought was her mistake, only to learn that the correct answer to the given task would have been that "it cannot be solved". Shortly thereafter the same teacher approached David with the request that he erase (!) the multiplication tables that he had been playfully drafting in his notebook, because "multiplication is not coming up until next term". Sadly, David obeyed and when the next term eventually came, he was handing in maths tests which contained ever more mistakes. There was no action whatsoever from the teacher to stop this deterioration—in fact, the teacher's comments became more rewarding as David got closer to acting like the other students in his class. Soon, he made it his own imperative "to not stand out" and, within several years, was among the lower-ranking students in terms of his maths grades. Ironically, his new maths teacher was now complaining that David was "not working in class, not asking any questions when given the chance, and not showing any initiative".

Being criticised into silence

A third way in which teachers may silence gifted students is by convincing them that they have nothing to say that would be particularly worth hearing and that their outputs or they themselves are flawed. This is especially the case when giftedness is expressed in a way that is at odds with the teacher's implicit theories: oftentimes the teacher will expect high-ability students to do their school work meticulously as required, with few or no mistakes; the same students, however, might be less concerned with the exact spelling or numbers, and more focused on the "big picture"—the underlying patterns and abstract ideas behind a text or scientific issue (e.g. Altaras, 2006). In such circumstances, the teacher may (choose to) insistently address the student's "weaknesses" (e.g. mistakes in orthography and calculation) and seldom or never reward their deep understanding or original treatment of a topic. Similarly, students who have a developed sense of humour and delight in playing with words—rather than simply following the instructions conveyed by them—may be scolded for being rude and disobedient and not at all appreciated for their wit (Gross, 1999). In short, the scenario described here is one where gifted students suffer criticism from the teacher until they learn to censor themselves.

This particular scenario applies to Nick, a third grader who was not very keen on producing the typical elementary school essays but could splendidly turn any material or personal experience into an original and humorous comic. Yet, rather than acknowledging this gift, his teacher's comments tended to focus solely on the linguistic or material errors in his written or spoken narrative, until eventually Nick stopped raising his hand in class. Luckily, he had not stopped making comics, one of which poignantly illustrated his frustration with his teacher's criticism and led his parents to seek out the help of an independent counsellor (psychologist). When they visited the school to enquire about Nick's deteriorating grades, his teacher had a ready explanation: Nick was just "too silent and withdrawn" and "not participating enough" in class.

Silencing the parent

Given the above scenarios, it is no wonder that many parents feel compelled to advocate for their gifted children. However, part of silencing gifted students is silencing their parents, too. Again, this may take different forms, one of which is disregarding or actively disbelieving the information that parents provide on their child's precociousness (Gross, 1999) and attempting to convince them that there is really nothing special about their child's cognitive development. Another way entails admitting that the child is precocious but suggesting that he/she is being pushed by the parents and would be better off without any meddling with the natural development (and hence without any special educational provisions).[1] A more sinister version of this scenario involves shaming or "deriding [the parents] for attempting to secure 'special treatment' for their children", which may even escalate to the level of "a vitriolic attack" on the parents (Silverman, 1994, as cited in Benbow & Stanley, 1996, p. 271).

A combination of the above-described silencing strategies was experienced by David's parents: initially, they were told by the teacher that David was "a normally developing child" who should not be exposed to any advanced curriculum. However, on the eve of a parent–teacher conference, the school had received an official report from the psychologist, confirming David's exceptional intellectual, and especially mathematical, abilities. When, during the conference, other parents were asking for some differentiation in maths, David's mother supported this initiative, pointing out both sides of the spectrum—the need to allow more

---

[1]As observed in Gross's studies, "No fewer than six of the 15 parents report that they have experienced various degrees of obstructiveness from teachers or school administrators who have countered requests for assistance by claiming that they themselves were parents of gifted children who succeeded academically without intervention" (p. 172).

time to the slower-progressing students, but also to provide additional and more complex tasks to the faster-working ones. She was careful not to use the label "gifted", but could still not avoid "sticking out like a sore thumb" (cf. VanTassel-Baska, 2009): Her utterance was, namely, the only one to elicit a direct reply from the teacher, who told her that "This is a regular school, not one for gifted children." Ironically, this was the same teacher who only a week earlier had described David as "normally developing" and advised against putting him in an advanced school. Looking back on this event, David's mother now feels that the teacher's response was instrumental in "shutting me up, by making it appear as if I were bragging about my son being gifted and demanding some special treatment for him. I cannot quite get over the fact that I remained silent instead of replying: 'Indeed, this is a regular school, and that means a school for all children, including those who are gifted.'"

A discussion of silencing giftedness

Putting the phenomenon into perspective: how bad is it?

Although the silencing of giftedness at school may not appear as dramatic as some other instances of silencing described in this volume, when gauging the severity of this phenomenon, there are several important things to note:

First, as with most forms of silencing, there is a fair amount of hostility, aggression, and violence attached to the silencing of giftedness, too. This has, for instance, been explicitly recognised in Gross's (2004) treatise on exceptionally gifted children: "A disturbing finding of this study is the *overt or veiled hostility* that the majority of the parents have experienced from teachers or school administrators" (p. 171, emphasis added). Essentially the same judgement is passed by giftedness researchers who use such terms as "neglect" and "abuse" to characterise the treatment of gifted students within the educational system (e.g. Benbow & Stanley, 1996).

Second, and following from the above, the students being silenced are getting hurt in the process (Benbow & Stanley, 1996), that is, they are suffering damage to both their academic and social-emotional development. School-related feelings of frustration and boredom are top of the list of the counselling needs of gifted pre-adolescents (Yoo & Moon, 2006), but may actually just be the tip of the iceberg, with more serious problems lurking underneath: for one thing, students whose talents are not recognised by their teachers are at risk of lower psychological well-being (Kroesbergen et al., 2016), and muting one's abilities for peer acceptance can diminish one's own sense of identity (Gross, 1998). Moreover, the silencing of gifted students can send them down a spiral of underachievement (cf. Altaras, 2006; Reis & McCoach, 2000), as illustrated by the case of David above or summarised in the words of another gifted child's parent: "We feel Richard underachieves because, after years of having his abilities suppressed at school, he has come to feel that achievement isn't really important" (Gross, 2004, p. 171). Ultimately, the damage may spread to other students, too: "If [our most rapid learners] are ignored, exploited, damaged, held back in their progress, or teased, the message we give to all children is that academic learning doesn't pay for anyone" (Kearney, 1993, as cited in Benbow & Stanley, 1996, p. 260).

Third, the silencing of gifted students stands as a paragon of absurdity and perversion, because what is silenced is the wish to learn—in a place meant for learning! Moreover, this is still happening at a time when schools are generally embracing inclusion and diversity, and increasingly tending to individual student needs (sometimes to the point of nurturing self-indulgence). Several authors had already noted this bias some two or three decades ago: Benbow and Stanley (1996) "wonder if Americans would allow *any other group* in our society to sustain and endure the abuse that highly achieving precocious children face on a daily basis in their schools" (p. 260, emphasis added), while Gross (1998) asks whether "the love of learning [has] now become 'the love that dare not speak its name'" (p. 171). Judging from the experiences of Vincent and David, these questions are relevant at the present time: evidently, the "special educational need" that the inclusive school of today may still be openly intolerant to is the need to know and learn more.

Fourth, the silencing of giftedness seems to be a global phenomenon (cf. Gaeke & Gross, 2008): The instances described above span at least three continents and four different educational systems, including the German and Serbian (examples from my own research experience), US-American (e.g. Benbow & Stanley, 1996), and Australian (e.g. Gross, 2004). Evidently—though paradoxically—the phenomenon of silencing giftedness is also native to economically prosperous, individualistic societies (Germany, USA, Australia), that tend to promote individual liberties and award individual achievements. Moreover, its global presence also implies that this phenomenon cannot be explained away by disadvantageous circumstances and/or specific cultural norms. How, then, are we to understand it? Why are gifted students being pervasively and ubiquitously silenced?

The reasons (and rationalisations) behind silencing giftedness

A good starting point to tackle this issue may be the following quote from Caroline Vincent—a participant in Gross's (2004) study—whose daughter, Jade, faced explicit denial of her giftedness by the teachers: "It's really disturbing when you realize what this sort of thing implies— that either these teachers have NO idea of the implications of such exceptionally high IQs, or that they are so determined to reduce the magnitude of the differences between the highly gifted kids and the others in the class that they will quite deliberately cut down the tall poppies to do so" (Gross, 2004, p. 173, emphasis in original). Thus, Jade's mother offers two possible answers to the above question: the first is—simple ignorance; the second—deliberately ignoring the needs of gifted students. But why would a teacher remain ignorant about this particular group of students or choose to ignore them?

Silencing out of convenience (and conventionality)

To answer this, the first thing to note is that teachers have been repeatedly found to prefer non-studious over studious students and athleticism over academic brilliance (Cramond & Martin, 1987; Lee et al., 2004). They also "seem to gravitate to students that are easier to handle"—who conform and follow along in class, accepting the teacher's instructions and authority unquestioningly (Kim, 2008, p. 236; see also Hernández-Torrano et al., 2013). Conversely, gifted students who express their curiosity and creativity in the classroom may be perceived as a nuisance or menace: they may threaten the teachers' self-esteem and authority, and awaken their fear of losing control of what is happening in the classroom, as well as of being redundant or even incompetent (cf. Gross, 1999, 2004). At the same time, these students require more investment and effort from the teacher: they want their questions answered and their abilities challenged, which, in an inclusive classroom, also means that the teacher must know how to differentiate and individualise instruction (e.g. Altaras Dimitrijević & Tatić Janevski, 2016). From this perspective, the silencing of gifted students appears as a convenient way to kill two birds with one stone—to save one's time and energy, and to save face as the indisputable authority in the classroom.

This, of course, requires a rationalisation, and this is where the Galton-inspired myth of the gifted thriving on their own, without any educational support, comes in quite handy. As observed by Moon (2009), this myth is "an attractive one for school personnel", because "[I]f the myth is true, teachers, principals, and superintendents have no responsibility to recognize the existence of this special population of students or to attempt to address their needs" (p. 274).

Silencing out of (political) conviction

However, the above quote from Jade's mother suggests that there is also the kind of deliberate silencing that seems to transcend the teacher's personal interests and follow a larger agenda—the agenda to "cut down the tall poppies", as the practice of holding back gifted students is commonly referred to in Australia (Gross, 1999). Again, two persistent myths about gifted students and gifted education serve to sustain this agenda.

It is bad for you to stand out. The first is the so-called "disharmony myth", entailing the stereotype of the academically brilliant, yet socially/emotionally troubled or troublesome individual. Though contradicting empirical research, this myth is still present among educators (Baudson & Preckel, 2013; Gaeke & Gross, 2008; Hernández-Torrano et al., 2013) and may lead them to believe that by silencing and slowing down giftedness they are actually helping the student adjust—or "come to his senses", as Vincent's teacher had put it. In other words, some teachers may make it their mission to "cure" their students of their giftedness, which would otherwise "consume" them and rob them of a "normal life" (or at least childhood).

It is wrong for you to stand out. The second myth is that fairness in the classroom can only be achieved by teaching all children the same way and that any curricular adjustments for gifted students are elitist, that is, a threat to social justice (Cooper, 2009; see also Baccassino & Pinnelli, 2023). According to Benbow and Stanley (1996), the myth of gifted education as elitist is based on a "changed meaning of equality", which more and more refers to our "striv[ing] for sameness in educational outcomes, rather than providing equal opportunities to develop differing potentialities" (p. 256). Consequently, enrichment may easily be misunderstood as "gifted students get[ting] richer while all others remain poor" (Gagné, 2007), and a well-intended educational policy like the *No Child Left Behind Act*[2] may quickly be misinterpreted to mean "no child allowed forward". Unfortunately, research has shown that teachers do, to a non-negligible extent, "buy into the myth of elitism concerning the education of the gifted" (Troxclair, 2013, p. 63; see also Jung, 2014; McCoach & Siegle, 2007). In fact, even those who personally hold a different view may decide to act according to the myth, realising that "programs for gifted students are not politically correct" (Benbow & Stanley, 1996, p. 271) and that—in the words of a principal cited by Gross (2004)—"[I]t would be 'political suicide' [...] to establish any differentiated program for the intellectually gifted students" (p. 4).

Sympathy for the teacher

In sum, several long-standing myths exist among educators and in society at large that uphold and rationalise the practice of silencing giftedness, the true goal of which might be to reduce workload, maintain control, preserve authority, and appease narcissistic injury and envy. In view of this, the key to ending this harmful practice may not simply be more formal training for the teachers, though the change can hardly start anywhere else but from working with educators (cf. Moon et al., 1997). Some authors have suggested that teachers be trained in creativity and nonconformity (Kim, 2008) or selected to work with gifted

---

[2] A US law of 2001, the full title of which serves to explain its main purpose: "An act to close the achievement gap with accountability, flexibility, and choice, so that no child is left behind."

students based on their expertise in and passion for the subject matter, as well as such personality characteristics as openness (Mills, 2003). The path that my colleagues and I are taking in an ongoing action research is listening to the—usually silent, but not so rare—voices of those "gifting" teachers who do (want to) individualise instruction for their gifted students, so as to learn from these teachers' experiences and speak out about how inclusive gifted education can be made to work.

References

Altaras, A. (2006). *Darovitost i podbacivanje (Giftedness and Underachievement)*. Pančevo-Beograd, Serbia: Mali Nemo, Institut za psihologiju & Centar za primenjenu psihologiju Društva psihologa Srbije.

Altaras Dimitrijević, A., & Tatić Janevski, S. (2016). *Obrazovanje učenika izuzetnih sposobnosti: Naučne osnove i smernice za školsku praksu (The Education of High-ability Students: Scientific Foundations and School-practice Guidelines)*. Beograd, Serbia: Zavod za unapređivanje obrazovanja i vaspitanja.

Baccassino, F., & Pinnelli, S. (2023). Giftedness and gifted education: A systematic literature review. *Frontiers in Education, 7*: 1073007.

Baudson, T. G., & Preckel, F. (2013). Teachers' implicit personality theories about the gifted: An experimental approach. *School Psychology Quarterly, 28*(1): 37–46.

Benbow, C. P., & Stanley, J. C. (1996). Inequity in equity: How "equity" can lead to inequity for high-potential students. *Psychology, Public Policy, and Law, 2*(2): 249–292.

Coleman, L. J., & Cross, T. L. (2000). Social-emotional development and the personal experience of giftedness. In: K. A. Heller, F. J. Mönks, R. J. Sternberg, & R. F. Subotnik (Eds.), *International Handbook of Giftedness and Talent* (2nd edn.) (pp. 203–212). New York: Elsevier.

Cooper, C. R. (2009). Myth 18: It is fair to teach all children the same way. *Gifted Child Quarterly, 53*(4): 283–285.

Cramond, B., & Martin, C. E. (1987). Inservice and preservice teachers' attitudes toward the academically brilliant. *Gifted Child Quarterly, 31*(1): 15–19.

Cross, T., Coleman, L., & Stewart, R. (1995). Psychosocial diversity of gifted adolescents: An exploration of the stigma of giftedness paradigm. *Roeper Review, 16*(1): 37–40.

Feldhusen, J. F., & Hoover, S. M. (1984). The gifted at risk in a place called school. *Gifted Child Quarterly, 28*(1): 9–11.

Gaeke, J. G., & Gross, M. U. M. (2008). Teachers' negative affect toward academically gifted students: An evolutionary psychological study. *Gifted Child Quarterly, 52*(3): 217–231.

Gagné, F. (2007). Ten commandments for academic talent development. *Gifted Child Quarterly, 51*(2): 93–118.

Galton, F. (1869). *Hereditary Genius: An Inquiry into Its Laws and Consequences.* London: Macmillan, 1892.

Gross, M. U. M. (1998). The "me" behind the mask: Intellectually gifted students and the search for identity. *Roeper Review, 20*(3): 167–174.

Gross, M. U. M. (1999). Small poppies: Highly gifted children in the early years. *Roeper Review, 21*(3): 207–214.

Gross, M. U. M. (2004). *Exceptionally Gifted Children* (2nd edn.). London: Routledge.

Händel, M., Vialle, W., & Ziegler, A. (2013). Student perceptions of high-achieving classmates. *High Ability Studies, 24*(2): 99–114.

Hernández-Torrano, D., Prieto, M. D., Ferrándiz, C., Bermejo, R., & Sáinz, M. (2013). Characteristics leading teachers to nominate secondary students as gifted in Spain. *Gifted Child Quarterly, 57*(3): 181–196.

Inbar, D. E. (1996). The free educational prison: Metaphors and images. *Educational Research, 38*(1): 77–92.

Jung, J. Y. (2014). Predictors of attitudes to gifted programs/provisions: Evidence from preservice educators. *Gifted Child Quarterly, 58*(4): 247–258.

Kim, K. H. (2008). Underachievement and creativity: Are gifted underachievers highly creative? *Creativity Research Journal, 20*(2): 234–242.

Kroesbergen, E. H., van Hooijdonk, M., van Viersen, S., Middel-Lalleman, M. M. N., & Reijnders, J. J. W. (2016). The psychological well-being of early identified gifted children. *Gifted Child Quarterly, 60*(1): 16–30.

Law on the fundamentals of the education system [Zakon o osnovama sistema obrazovanja i vaspitanja]. *Službeni glasnik RS*, br. 72/09, 52/11 и 55/13.

Lee, S.-Y., Cramond, B., & Lee, J. (2004). Korean teachers' attitudes toward academic brilliance. *Gifted Child Quarterly, 48*(1): 42–53.

Lee, S.-Y., Olszewski-Kubilius, P., & Turner Thompson, D. (2012). Academically gifted students' perceived interpersonal competence and peer relationships. *Gifted Child Quarterly, 56*(2): 90–104.

McCoach, D. B., & Siegle, D. (2007). What predicts teachers' attitudes toward the gifted? *Gifted Child Quarterly, 51*(3): 246–255.

Mills, C. J. (2003). Characteristics of effective teachers of gifted students: Teacher background and personality styles of students. *Gifted Child Quarterly, 47*(4): 272–281.

Moon, S. M. (2009). Myth 15: High-ability students don't face problems and challenges. *Gifted Child Quarterly, 53*(4): 274–276.

Moon, S. M., Kelly, K. R., & Feldhusen, J. F. (1997). Specialized counseling services for gifted youth and their families. A needs assessment. *Gifted Child Quarterly, 41*(1): 16–25.

Myers, M. (2015, September 21). Roger Waters on "Another Brick in the Wall": Roger Waters discusses the making of "Another Brick in the Wall, Part 2". *The Wall Street Journal*, https://wsj.com/articles/roger-waters-on-another-brick-in-the-wall-1442855084

Reis, S. M., & McCoach, D. B. (2000). The underachievement of gifted students: What do we know and where do we go? *Gifted Child Quarterly, 44*(3): 152–170.

Sternberg, R. J., & Davidson, J. E. (2005). *Conceptions of Giftedness* (2nd edn.). Cambridge: Cambridge University Press.

Troxclair, D. A. (2013). Preservice teacher attitudes toward giftedness. *Roeper Review, 35*: 58–64.

VanTassel-Baska, J. (2009). Myth 12: Gifted programs should stick out like a sore thumb. *Gifted Child Quarterly, 53*(4): 266–268.

Winner, E. (1996). *Gifted Children: Myths and Realities*. New York: Basic Books.

Yoo, J. E., & Moon, S. M. (2006). Counseling needs of gifted students: An analysis of intake forms at a university-based counseling center. *Gifted Child Quarterly, 50*(1): 52–61.

CHAPTER 8

Censorship and silencing artistic creativity

Aleksandar Dimitrijević

> *Everyone had someone to cry over, but you had to cry silently,*
> *under your blanket, so that no one would see. Everyone feared*
> *everyone else, and the sorrow oppressed and suffocated us (...)*
> *So many unsaid things collect in the soul, so much exhaustion and*
> *irritation lie as a heavy burden on the psyche. And you must, you*
> *must unburden your spiritual world or risk a collapse. Sometimes*
> *you feel like screaming, but you control yourself and just babble*
> *some nonsense.*
>
> Dmitri Shostakovich

Athenians prohibited theatrical depictions of the then-contemporary contents that were not already known to all the spectators. Christians forbade theatre altogether as a form of Dionysian cult, as well as countless books and paintings. Islam shuns presenting any human figures. Shakespeare, Mozart, and Michelangelo, to name only a few of the greatest, had to wait for their works to be approved by the sources of higher power. Countless films have remained unreleased or can be seen only by limited audiences even today. Different novels were found unacceptable throughout history and are censored even in the allegedly most democratic countries of today. A mere 500 metres from where I am writing these words, Nazis burnt 25,000 books before 40,000 witnesses (Green & Karolides, 2005, pp. 11, 67–68), including the works by Heine, Freud, Mann, *All Quiet on the Western Front*, and many others, only four months after they had come to power in 1933.

Silencing via official impositions upon artistic or scientific creativity has been with us almost since the dawn of civilisation. No ideology likes uninhibited creativity. The more totalitarian its basic tenets are, the stricter its censorship mechanisms will be. We call it totalitarianism because it strives for absolute control over everything. All decisions come from only one centre, whether about the economy, education, civil liberties, life and death, war or peace. And as if this were not enough, they must also control the imagination. They have to tell everyone how to imagine their gods, how to propose marriage, what to play with other children, and what to dream about at night. Possibly most importantly, they want to decide about how trauma will be expressed and processed, knowing that arts play a crucial role here (Dimitrijević, 2020). Until the imagination is enslaved, people are never entirely silenced.

Some illustrations of the totalitarian censorship of the arts in twentieth-century Europe

European totalitarian regimes of the twentieth century were led by two failed artists who had no political ambitions in their early years. However, as soon as they fortified their respective positions of undisputed power, they both made fateful decisions about artworks and artists alike.

In the West, it was an aspiring painter who believed he had something to say about Wagner's music, and initiated, organised, and executed a world war and the Shoah. Countless influential intellectuals were murdered, exiled, or incarcerated during the twelve years of his rule—a devastation Europe will never recover from. As many as 2500 authors left Germany immediately in 1933 (Green & Karolides, 2005, p. 67), like Einstein, and others only to save their children, like Freud; some had their German citizenship revoked, like Remarque and Georg Grosz;[1] some decided never to return, like Thomas Mann. The music of Jewish composers was forbidden, including Mendelssohn Bartholdy and Mahler, who had both converted. Everything subsumed under the expression "degenerate art", including expressionist and secessionist paintings, was confiscated and hidden at best, while often burned. Hitler and his propaganda machinery constantly repeated what kind of art they were willing to permit and support. These had to be contributions that praised German history, mythology, language, and the imagined uniqueness of the German "race", health, optimism, and (eternal) superiority.

In the East, millions have died under the despotic rule of a former fledgling poet who had grown up in a seminary in what is now Georgia. Everyone feared him, and he was directly responsible for the deaths of millions whom he led to starvation, sent to gulags in Siberia, or ordered assassinated. Yet, probably no one feared him as much as, on the one side, poets and artists and, on the other, priests and monks. In the twenty-five years of his dictatorship, he had many of them tortured and killed, and many had to write, film, or compose precisely what he wanted and how he wanted it. There were 700 writers at the Congress of Writers' Union in 1934, but only fifty of them survived until the Congress in 1954 (MacDonald, 2006, p. 394, n. 29).[2]

On May 7, 1926, secret police agents raided Mikhail Bulgakov's apartment and confiscated the only two existing copies of *The Heart of a Dog*, "unpublished for censorship reasons",[3] and three notebooks of the author's diaries (Shentalinsky, 1996, pp. 72ff.). None of these were to be returned for years, despite the author's repeated official appeals. Once he finally got them back, he immediately tore the diaries apart and burnt them. Yet, we can read them today because the police photographed them and had them typed. No one was aware of this for the next seventy years, neither was Bulgakov when he wrote the now famous

---

[1] It is interesting that Grosz's paintings were included in the Nazi exhibition "Degenerate art", only to be censored again in the US and Italy in the 1950s (Green & Karolides, 2005, p. 217).

[2] These are, of course, miniscule numbers in comparison with the whole country: two million "political prisoners" died in the gulag only in 1937–1938 (MacDonald, 2006, p. 399, n. 79), and in 1941, every fifth person worked as a slave (ibid., p. 146).

[3] This is a quote from the interrogation report dated September 22, 1926.

line "Manuscripts don't burn". To study Soviet art means to work in the archives of Lubyanka, the secret police Moscow headquarters. If we focus only on the most important names, everyone was interrogated there: Babel, Blok, Bulgakov, Demidov, Florenski, Mandelshtam, Pilnyak, Platonov, Sholokhov, Shostakovich, and even the hero of the October Revolution, Maxim Gorky himself.

Musical geniuses like Rachmaninov and Stravinsky decided never to return. At the same time, Nabokov, Chagall, and Tarkovsky[4] were forced to leave if they wanted to preserve their authenticity and creative liberties, which was also the case with countless performing artists of the highest level.[5] Solzhenitsyn was forcefully exiled in 1974 having spent eight years in Siberia, and his cardinal sin, like that of Boris Pasternak, was being awarded the Nobel Prize for literature. Many of their works, and other most important Soviet novels, were smuggled and published abroad.

Many were never arrested, but they could not publish anything for decades, including the great poet Anna Akhmatova. Her silence was secured by sending her husband and son to a camp so they could be killed if she ever spoke (MacDonald, 2006, p. 116; Shentalinsky, 1996). Pasternak spent years translating and writing nothing of his own, yet Olga Ivinskaya, his lover and the true inspiration for the character of Larisa Antipova, was sent to the gulag in 1950 together with her fourteen-year-old daughter, and both were arrested again almost immediately after the poet died in 1960 (Finn & Couvée, 2014).[6] Shostakovich also always had a close relative somewhere in Siberia.

It all ended even more tragically for some others. Gumilyov was shot as early as 1921 (before Stalin's dictatorship). The literary critics Averbakh and Pilnyak, and the theologian and polymath Florensky were shot in 1937. Babel and Meyerhold, the theatre revolutionary,

---

[4]Tarkovsky shot almost one-third of *Stalker* before it became evident that the film he was given had a layer of green, and all of the material had to be thrown away. He started from scratch, but when his masterpiece was ready, it could only be seen in three cinemas in Moscow, a city of 10 million people (Tarkovsky, 1989).

[5]Including Shostakovich's son Maxim who defected to West Germany in 1982 and later asked for political asylum in the US.

[6]Finn and Couvée, 2014, also provide compelling evidence about the propaganda use of *Dr. Zhivago* by the CIA against the Soviet Union.

in 1940. Daniil Kharms in 1942. Osip Mandelstam died in a camp in 1938. Yesenin committed suicide in 1925, Mayakovsky in 1930, Tsvetaeva in 1941, and Fadeev in 1956.

The tyrant took so much care that he observed, controlled, and decided himself, despite all the other things he had to control and/ or destroy. In April 1930, Stalin himself called Mikhail Bulgakov,[7] for which there were two more witnesses, and soon after Bulgakov was appointed the director of Moscow Art Theatre. In June 1934, he called Pasternak to enquire whether Mandelstam was a great poet (Shentalinsky, 1996, p. 184). He also called Shostakovich on March 16, 1948, pretending not to know that his music was banned.[8]

In some cases, the problems stemmed from individual incidents. For instance, Stalin did not like the first part of *Lady Macbeth from Mzensk* (luckily, he left the performance before the protagonists are arrested and have to walk to the prison in Siberia).[9] Mandelstam had composed a poem against the dictator, which was discovered although he never wrote it down but only recited it, whispering, to the trusted ones. Rostropovich sheltered Solzhenitsyn after the latter's return from the gulags.

There needed to be no incidents whatsoever for someone to be destroyed. One interrogator said to Pavel Florensky: "Our job is to anticipate. Do they expect us to wait until someone has committed a crime and only then punish them? No, that's no good" (Shentalinsky, 1996, p. 119). As the historian Orlando Figes corroborated from various sources (2007), everyone in the Soviet Union "was in effect placed in a solitary confinement" (MacDonald, 2006, p. 146), as the secret police had unlimited power.[10]

---

[7] Stalin also allegedly saw Bulgakov's *Days of the Turbins* fifteen times (Shentalinsky, 1996, p. 88).

[8] Maxim never forgot how his mother was listening to this conversation on another telephone in their apartment, and even he, still a boy, got to hear Stalin's voice (in Ardov, 2004, pp. 70–72).

[9] Shostakovich (1981, p. 104) described "Stalin's envy of someone else's fame", but it seems impossible to know whether he was right about this.

[10] For an attempt to disentangle the roles of loneliness and solitude in artistic creativity, see Dimitrijević, 2022.

The great actor, playwright, and novelist Mikhail Bulgakov wrote in his diary that he should better "... hold my tongue in the hopes that in future I would again be allowed to speak" (October 26, 1923), and repeated this in public and personal documents, like his letter to the Government of the USSR of March 28, 1930, where he stated: "... I am doomed to the lifetime of silence in the USSR," or one to Maxim Gorky, "Everything has been banned, I am ruined, persecuted and totally alone" (September 6, 1929). Beginning in January 1922, Bulgakov repeatedly used expressions like these: starving, in debt, cancerous tissue, depression and nostalgia, nothing to wear, completely broken man, banned, taken off, unemployed, demonised, refused, removed, doomed, unacceptable, material catastrophe, extreme exhaustion, persecution, final ruin, destitution, homelessness and death, neurasthenia, panic attacks, heart-related anxiety, insomnia, hunted. And he eloquently described his desperation at being silenced: "condemned to silence" (January 16, 1930); "reduced to silence; for a writer this is equivalent to death" (February 21, 1930); "condemned to a lifetime of silence" (March 28, 1930); "falling silent ... And if a real writer has fallen silent, he will perish" (May 30, 1931). His worries that because he was "unable to work in this atmosphere of absolute hopelessness, my annihilation as a writer will be followed by complete and definite physical collapse" (letter to the head of the main committee for the arts, July 30, 1929) ultimately proved correct, as he was to die in 1940, at the age of just forty-eight, ill, hungry, frozen, and unrecognised. A fully uncensored version of *Master and Margarita*, his life's work, was only published in 1973.

More importantly for our topic, at two moments, in 1934 and 1948, whole doctrines were developed with the basic purpose of silencing individual artistic creativity. The term "socialist realism" first appeared in a literary journal in 1932, and the authorship was later attributed to Stalin himself (MacDonald, 2006, p. 119), although some believe it came from Zhdanov or Gorky. Official definitions of the term are totally obscure and hardly understandable: "the aesthetic face of Marxist truth", "portraying reality in its revolutionary development as though looking at the present from the future golden age", or "the artist's justified emotion in the face of the real mass heroism of the struggle for socialism" (MacDonald, 2006, p. 120), or "an all-healing feeling of the ultimate rightness of reality" (in Behrman, 2010, p. 56). General Zhdanov, who ruthlessly imposed it, claimed that "socialist realism, the basic method of Soviet artistic literature and literary criticism, demands truthfulness from the artist and an historically concrete portrayal of reality in its revolutionary development" (in Behrman, 2010, p. 56).

The aim of it all was "to assimilate art as soon as possible into the general propaganda effort" and create "music for the millions" (MacDonald, 2006, p. 121).[11] The requirement was that all art had to be understandable to everyone, while the whole truth was that art had to influence and indoctrinate everyone. At the same time, the worst enemy was named formalism, art that followed purely aesthetic principles, individualism, and introspection. By no means was art supposed to express any pessimism.[12] Soviet psychiatry came up with a mental disorder named "metaphysical intoxication", applicable to all those who asked whether Communism was indeed the final answer to all the questions (Fulford et al., 1993).

As an example to others, Stalin used none other than Shostakovich, the most important and popular Soviet composer, and his 1936 attack on Shostakovich changed the Soviet cultural scene forever (Behrman, 2010, p. 61). The official outlet of the Communist Party, *Pravda*, published an article "Muddle instead of music", on January 28, 1936.[13] Shostakovich's incredibly popular opera *Lady Macbeth from Mzensk* was described as a "cacophonous and pornographic insult to the Soviet people" a mere two days after Stalin had stormed out of one performance. The article concluded that "things may end very badly" for *tovarish* Shostakovich. The composer immediately lost all his friends, prospects, and positions, was interrogated, and expected arrest and deportation. He later (1981, p. 86)

---

[11] Musical geniuses, of course, understood everything thoroughly. Shostakovich said, "In examining the works of a young composer, there is too much discussion about whether, for example, the music adequately conveys that the collective farm has fulfilled its plan by one hundred per cent" (in MacDonald, 2006, p. 122), and Prokofiev that "what people here dub formalism is actually a simple matter of not understanding something on first hearing" (in Wilson, 2006, p. 134).

[12] The epitome of this was *Hamlet* and both the play and the character were frequently used as means of criticising "formalist artists".

[13] It is still uncertain who wrote the article. Some historians think that it was Zhdanov (Roseberry, 1986, pp. 85, 120), while Shostakovich (1981, p. 86) believed that it was Stalin himself.

recalled that if his music was ever played, it was announced in a special way: "Today there is a concert by enemy of the people Shostakovich."

While the world suffered during the Second World War, most Soviet artists experienced this period as an intermezzo. Only threatening rumours were heard: "As soon as we are done with the Allies we'll put your Shostakovich under our thumbnail!" (Shostakovich, 1981, p. 105). And indeed, already in August 1946, Zhdanov attacked Akhmatova and Zoshchenko, then turned to cinema and theatre (Behrman, 2010, p. 79), claiming that

> the task of Soviet literature is to aid the state to educate the youth correctly and to meet their demands, to rear a new generation strong and vigorous, believing in their cause, fearing no obstacles and ready to overcome all obstacles. Consequently any preaching of ideological neutrality, of political neutrality, of "art for art's sake" is alien to Soviet literature and harmful to the interests of the Soviet people and the Soviet state. (in Green & Karolides, 2005, p. 667)

In January 1948, it was the composers' turn. Shostakovich, Prokofiev, Khachaturian, Weinberg, and many others were no longer permitted to teach, perform, and publish. "Zhdanov announced, 'The Central Committee of Bolsheviks demands beauty and refinement from music,' And he added that the goal of music was to give pleasure, while our music was crude and vulgar, and listening to it undoubtedly destroyed the psychological and physiological balance of a man" (Shostakovich, 1981, p. 111).

Socialist realism silenced artists to such a degree that the poet Osip Mandelstam wrote that "… ten steps away no one hears our speeches …" (in Roseberry, 1986, p. 135). Those not murdered suffered profound emotional disturbances: "An existence like this leaves its mark. We all became slightly unbalanced mentally—not exactly ill, but not normal either: suspicious, mendacious, confused and inhibited in our speech, at the same time putting on a show of adolescent optimism" (Nadezhda Mandelstam, in MacDonald, 2006, p. 135). Shostakovich (1981) later admitted this condition "… oppressed me, it deprived me of the will to compose [p. 103] … I was near to suicide" (p. 89). Stalin's second wife killed herself, and having seen the consequences of mass famine in Ukraine in 1934, Pasternak could not sleep for an entire year (MacDonald, 2006, p. 117). Probably the most eloquent account of the situation can be found in the suicide note written by the president of the Soviet Writers' Union, Alexander Fadeyev, on May 13, 1956: "I do not see the possibility of going on living, since art, to which I have dedicated my life, has been ruined by self-confidently ignorant leadership of the party, and can no longer now be repaired. The best cadres of literature … have been physically destroyed, or have perished thanks to the criminal connivance of those in power; the best people of literature died before their time" (in MacDonald, 2006, p. 393, n. 5).[14]

The only thing still allowed was propaganda, exaggerated optimism about the Soviet present and future: "It's as if someone were beating you with a stick and saying, 'your business is rejoicing, your business is rejoicing', and you rise, shakily and go marching off muttering 'Our business is rejoicing, our business is rejoicing …'" (Shostakovich, 1981, pp. 140, 183).

Yet, not everyone agreed. Anna Akhmatova remembered a random but potentially life-changing encounter:

> I spent seventeen months waiting in prison queues in Leningrad. One day, there was a woman standing behind me, her lips blue with cold, who, of course, had never in her life heard my name. Jolted out of the torpor characteristic of all of us, she said into my ear (everyone whispered there) "Could one ever describe this?" And I answered, "I can." It was then that something like a smile slid across what had previously been just a face.

Akhmatova's *Requiem* bears witness that she never lost the awareness that "one hundred million voices shout" through her "tortured mouth".

Composers could use the greater ambiguity of musical expression (compared to verbal statements or visual portraiture) to express even the most forbidden. The most famous example of this is Shostakovich's

---

[14] It is important to note that Fadeyev killed himself after being reported to the secret police by his fellow writer and alleged friend Mikhail Sholokhov.

Tenth Symphony, which premiered in 1953, the year of Stalin's death.[15] Its second movement, strangely brief at about four minutes, especially after the very long and abstract first movement, and full of brutal passages, represents Stalin. The third movement, however, is obviously a self-portrait, as it revolves around the tones D–Es–C–H, Shostakovich's musical signature, where the initial of his last name was spelled out in the German orthography (sch). Musicologists had problems interpreting this movement, but it seems to me that it was later described in words. Reminiscing about his life, Shostakovich spoke of his feelings after the premiere of *Lady Macbeth from Mzensk*:

> Before the opera I was a boy who might have been spanked, and later I was a state criminal, always under observation, always under suspicion. But at that moment everything was comparatively fine. Or to be more accurate, everything seemed fine. (1981, p. 84)

In the third movement of the *Tenth*, the D–Es–C–H signature first appears high in the oboes and violins, very playfully ("… a boy …"). After variations, it repeats as a waltz, announced in French horns, bassoons, and oboes, and executed in *forte* played *tutti*, to portray the almost exuberant strength of a young man for whom "everything was comparatively fine". However, this is almost immediately followed by harsh strikes in the percussions, alternating with the D–Es–C–H in violins in *crescendo* but in diminishing scales (just like the composer must have experienced the aforementioned *Pravda* article). The finale of this brutal torture against the artist who has just experienced a moment of triumph but now must run in despair is given to flutes, which repeat D–Es–C–H twice, until the movement ends with the third repetition, in piccolo, played *staccato*, as if to say, "You can try to break me as much as you want. I will, no matter how small I could be, continue expressing my identity even with my last dying breath." This feeling haunts the listener until the finale of the fourth movement (and the whole symphony)

---

[15] "The thaw" that came about after the tyrant's death was undoubtedly an enormous relief. Many forget, however, the importance of Zhdanov's death in 1948 at fifty-two, at the height of his purges.

when D–Es–C–H returns *fortissimo* and *tutti* to triumph finally over the dead dictator and his censors. The Stalin motif no longer appears, as the tyrant is dead and the creator has outlived him. Just as Rudolf Barshai, Shostakovich's student and the prominent violist and conductor, would later say in an interview, "In the future, historians will write, 'Stalin, important political figure from the era of Shostakovich'".[16]

Censorship in the country between East and West

Yugoslavia, a socialist country outside the Communist bloc, with its own rock'n'roll scene, comics, and an animated film that won the Oscar, enjoyed more freedom than Stalin would ever allow it. The premiere of Beckett's *Waiting for Godot* and several films that did not idealise the role of communist partisans in the Second World War were enough for the authorities to change the rules. During the brief relief in 1967–1968 (Vučetić, 2016, p. 268), Yugoslavian films flourished and won international acclaim. But many of the best ones belonged to what was called the New Film, or the Black Wave—the portrayal of challenges or unfulfilled promises of the society, without optimism and "beautifying". Then started the "restalinisation".

In 1969, a court case was opened against Želimir Žilnik over his film *Early Works*. Possibly because Žilnik was born in a concentration camp in Niš, his mother was executed by the German army and his father, killed in 1944, was posthumously decorated as a Hero of the People, the court did not rule against an artist for the first time (Vučetić, 2016. pp. 278–280). However, very soon after this, Žilnik was kicked out of the Communist Party and was forbidden from working as a film director (ibid., p. 282).

Dušan Makavejev was a renowned film director and editor to whose work many studies were devoted (e.g. Mortimer, 2009). When I started working at the University of Belgrade, I learned that many people still remembered Makavejev as a psychology student, although more than thirty years had passed. He was described to me as "frighteningly intelligent" and "the best student in ten generations".

---

[16] This refers to the documentary film *The Note*, available at https://youtube.com/watch?v=JXaKlf3y8Y4&t=2399s. The quoted sentence begins at 30′47″.

I believe that his psychological background is evident in both his method of filmmaking and his choice of topics. Starting with his *Innocence Unprotected*, which won him the Silver Bear Extraordinary Prize of the Jury at the 1968 Berlin Film Festival, Makavejev applied a highly effective and often hilarious blend of documentary materials and feature films, expert interviews and outrageous improvisations.

Makavejev's second film was even more ambitious and bore an enigmatic title, *WR: Mysteries of the Organism*.[17] He had decided to resurrect the life and work of Wilhelm Reich (hence the "WR" in the title).[18] Makavejev travelled to the US to interview Reich's son, patients, collaborators, and neighbours. He repeated and dramatised Reich's thesis that economic liberation had to be followed by sexual liberation.

The film was finalised in 1971 and initially survived the ideological commission. It was then screened before a test audience in Novi Sad in January 1972 (for details, see Vučetić, 2016, pp. 295ff.). It is important to note that the purpose of this was not to see whether the film would be popular and bring in money, as with test audiences in the West, but whether workers, the proletariat, Communist Party members, would also approve of it ideologically, regardless of their educational level or aesthetic preferences and sophistication. In this specific case, the opinion was asked of a large group of Second World War veterans. They found it offensive that a shot of Stalin's portrait followed immediately after a scene in which an erect penis was shown.[19] Makavejev then, in an interview given to foreign press while he was abroad, called the test audience members Stalinists. They sued him, and he did get sentenced and did not return to Yugoslavia for almost twenty years. And although the film had been very well received at the Cannes Film Festival, it was banned in Yugoslavia for the next sixteen years.

Also, in the 1970s, several other film directors of similar persuasion were blacklisted and punished. The trigger for this was a film made as a student exam submission (*Plastic Jesus* by Lazar Stojanović), which

---

[17] It is very telling that Makavejev was a member of that very "censorship commission (L. 14)" that, among others, assessed his own films (Vučetić, 2016, p. 291).

[18] For more details about Reich, see Chapter 9, this volume.

[19] Interestingly, only two years later, the new Yugoslavian constitution included the crime of "endangering of friendly relations with other states".

was never shown publicly. The censors thought that the film was critical of Josip Broz, the lifelong president of Yugoslavia, and Stojanović, another former psychology student, was expelled from the Communist Party and sent to prison for three years (1972–1975), after which he was allowed to leave the country. The film premiered only in 1990.

But it did not end there. In 1973, Stojanović's university mentor was fired, and his passport was confiscated. The mentor was none other than Aleksandar Petrović, one of the foremost film directors in Europe at that time, with various accolades at the Cannes and Venice festivals, two Oscar and one Golden Globe nominations. Petrović would then be forced to work abroad, and many of his films would be banned in Yugoslavia.[20]

Almost immediately after the film directors, the trouble began for the best storyteller and novelist of the younger generation, Danilo Kiš. Initially a widely acclaimed, awarded, and translated author, in 1976, Kiš published a collection of short stories, *A Tomb for Boris Davidovich*. His early works often dealt with the Shoah and the figure of his father, who was, as a Hungarian Jew, murdered in Auschwitz when the future author was still a boy. Kiš now turned to concentration camps in the USSR, noticing, during his several years' work at the universities of Strasbourg and Bordeaux, that many left-oriented intellectuals in France did not believe these camps ever existed.

No official body condemned or banned the book, but several persons accused Kiš of plagiarism. Texts were published in Zagreb and Belgrade that claimed Kiš had stolen other people's ideas and descriptions, that he had no right to write about the gulag as he had never experienced it himself, that he merely repeated Solzhenytzin ... Among the authors of these pamphlets were some very influential persons from the literary world and university professors, all reasonably well-established members of the Communist Party.

---

[20] It is fascinating that, while in exile, Petrović felt very inspired by the writings of Mikhail Bulgakov. No more than five years after the novel was first published, he adapted it for the screen and directed *The Master and Margarita*, which was almost immediately banned in Yugoslavia. Petrović also wrote a script for *Heart of a Dog* but never managed to shoot it, and he dramatised both works for the theatre.

As a passionate reader of Borges, Kiš applied the intertextual approach in each of his stories, quoting, inventing sources, events, and persons, mixing facts and fiction playfully. This writing style may have been new even for literary critics and university literature professors in Yugoslavia. But they likely only used a formal complaint as an excuse because they hated the content. All seven stories in the collection are related to Communism—the October Revolution, Stalinist purges, and the Spanish Civil War—and all are very critical. For example, one portrayed the fabrication of Soviet reality for a foreign delegation investigating civil liberties. The central one describes a hero of the revolution (Trotsky?) who falls out of grace, goes through a series of mock trials, and agrees to confess to anything after the prosecutors start killing one young man every evening and putting the blame on Boris Davidovich.

The book was a best-seller, published in more than thirty editions in Serbo-Croat and translated into more than twenty languages, with five English editions, four German and Spanish editions, and sometimes more than one translation to a certain language. It was soon dramatised and often performed in theatres nationwide and abroad.

Although envy or resistance to current literary trends could be significant sources of this case of silencing, the ideological one must have been at work as well, and Kiš referred to them repeatedly. He was the only artist mentioned in this chapter who got the opportunity to respond explicitly. In 1978, he published *The Anatomy Lesson*, a polemical book of essays that also got translated into many languages, and in which he elaborated his poetics and attacked those who had attacked him. This led to lawsuits, and in 1981 Kiš moved to Paris permanently. He was not silenced in the form of arrest or prohibition, but his literary reputation and integrity were attacked, and he chose exile to be able to focus on his writing. He later died at the age of fifty-four, a serious contender for the Nobel Prize for literature that he never got to win.

Examples of contemporary non-ideological censorship

There are also countless examples of contemporary censorship of artistic creativity unrelated to totalitarian ideologies (although some might become almost totalitarian soon). They are not motivated by religious notions (as described in this volume, Chapter 6) or by one political ideology which wants to silence all others—although such examples obviously exist as well[21]—but partly by those advocating against pornography and primarily by financial interests. In recent years, an informal movement called "cancel culture" has become very prominent in several Western countries, and it seems that here "cancel" is a euphemism for "censor".

In 1822, a statue of Achilles, placed in Hyde Park, London, had to have a leaf added to it to cover the genitalia (Green & Karolides, 2005, p. 3). But one can wonder whether things have changed with the passage of time. At the moment, as I am writing this at the beginning of April 2023, one piece of news has received international attention amid wars, climate change, and bank collapse. A school principal, not a celebrity, from a small town in Florida, USA, which most of us will never visit, had to resign. The point of broad interest has been the reason for her resignation. In her school, twelve-year-old children were shown Michelangelo's *David* and Botticelli's *Birth of Venus* in art class. Their parents considered this inappropriate and pornographic. Scholars remind us that copies of the statue have already suffered the same destiny, from Florence itself in 1504 to California and Sydney (Green & Karolides, 2005, p. 140), as have the copies of the *Venus de Milo* in Germany, Hungary, Kuwait, and the US (ibid., pp. 635–636). What is specific in the case of the Florida principal is that the demand for her resignation is a message that exposure to such works of art must not be repeated with future generations of students, making this demand not just a simple act of pressure but also an act of censorship of school programmes and materials.

Unfortunately, this is only the most recent example of this tendency, the proverbial tip of the iceberg. In the US, there is an organisation focused on raising public awareness of the problem of censoring books in public libraries. Every year, hundreds of people

---

[21] Some examples of this could be the treatment of *Diaries* by the former English government minister Richard Crossman, or reports of journalist Julian Assange or former agent Edward Snowden, as well as the McCarthyism, Watergate scandal, and US President Nixon's attempts to intimidate and control the press. Apart from this, some US states have censored Darwin's theory of evolution from being taught in schools. When it comes to the World Press Freedom Index for 2023, all of the highest places go to northern European EU members, while Germany is 21st, the UK 26th, and the US 45th (https://rsf.org/en/index).

complain that certain books should not be publicly available, and among them are elite twentieth-century novels, like Huxley's *Brave New World*, Kazantzakis's *The Last Temptation of Christ*, Lawrence's *Lady Chatterley's Lover*, Salinger's *The Catcher in the Rye*, Steinback's *The Grapes of Wrath*, and various books by Maya Angelou, Margaret Atwood, Ernest Hemingway, Stephen King, Henry Miller, Toni Morrison, Kurt Vonnegut, and Richard Wright. To prove all of the author's points, Orwell's *1984* is also on the list. More surprisingly, so is Whitman's *Leaves of Grass, the* classic of American literature. In the UK, a similar list also included books by Sartre and Voltaire. Among the reasons for these complaints, the most frequent ones are related to racism and offence to LGBTQI communities, even when books are 150 years old.

Especially criticised was Mark Twain's *The Adventures of Huckleberry Finn*. When it was published in 1884, many wanted it banned for it was "couched in the language of a rough, ignorant dialect", for its "systematic use of bad grammar and an employment of inelegant expressions", "trash of the vilest sort", and "a series of experiences that are certainly not elevating" (in Green & Karolides, 2005, p. 4). But over the last decades, the focus of criticism has been the representation of enslaved people and the use of racial slurs, so some editions now change Twain's phrasing.

In England, the Director of Public Prosecutions throughout the 1920s, Archibald Bodkin, saw Freud's works "as filth and threatened its publishers, Allen and Unwin, with prosecution unless they restricted its circulation to doctors, lawyers, and university dons, all of whom had to give their names and addresses when purchasing the book" (Green & Karolides, 2005, p. 62). Bodkin described Joyce's *Ulysses* as "indescribable filth" and "sent policemen to interrogate the critic F. R. Leavis, then a young Cambridge lecturer, who had requested the publishers in Paris to send him a copy for teaching purposes. The police duly infiltrated Leavis's lectures, with special orders to count the number of women present" (ibid.). English customs officers regularly confiscated copies of the novel for years, and court decisions regulated its distribution in the US.

Roald Dahl and J. K. Rowling faced similar problems because (some of) their books for children include portrayals of witches and magic.

There are always dozens of groups that advocate for stricter censorship in the US and many in the UK. The "American Family Association", "Coalition for Better Television", and "Citizens for Decent Literature" are just some of them. They try to influence the government of the US to introduce new laws and regulations and constantly campaign to boycott sponsors and advertisers of programmes they do not support (Green & Karolides, 2005, p. 13). Even before Al Gore became the vice president of the US, his wife, Tipper, founded a commission to make pop music free of "pornographic" material.[22] She certainly did not expect her most articulate opponent to be Frank Zappa, the most versatile American musician ever. Zappa testified before the US Senate in 1985, always defending the right to artistic expression (Zappa & Occhiogrosso, 1999), and even considered running for president in 1996. Still, some warning labels were introduced, similar to those in the film industry, and some level of censorship still persists.

On October 1, 1993, stand-up comedian Bill Hicks was invited to the show hosted by David Letterman, and he recorded a seven-minute routine with the audience present. Yet it was cut out of the show. Although Hicks had become famous for his relentless criticism of religious and political institutions, this time he was censored for the content deemed offensive to the show's sponsors (True, 2002). The television network or the show producers feared the jokes could hurt their income and censored them without hesitation. Still, that is much better than the multiple arrests and jail sentences Lenny Bruce had to face for the contents of his comedy acts thirty years earlier, and George Carlin's "comedic essay" about seven dirty words one is not allowed to say on television.

The expression "film industry" is justified for many reasons, only one of them being related to the ownership: while artworks belong to their authors (even if they are dedicated to someone, including a patron), films belong to their producers, who make final decisions about their content, form, casting, or ending. The abuse of this power became public knowledge with the "Me Too" movement when many actresses

---

[22] Much earlier, Billie Holiday's tragic demise was at least accelerated by the unofficial prohibition of her song "Strange Fruit" to the lyrics by Abel Meeropol, which refers to the lynching and hanging of African Americans done by the Ku Klux Klan.

testified to blackmail and sexual abuse they were exposed to by some super-powerful film producers.

Regarding the artistic process, it probably started with *The Golden Age* by Louis Bunuel and Salvador Dali, which premiered in Paris in 1931 but was so savagely attacked by various right-wing groups that it was closed down after six days, to be seen again only in 1981 (Green & Karolides, 2005, p. 7). Tennessee Williams and Elia Kazan jointly made several films, almost all of which were shortened under the pressure of the so-called Legion of Decency. The censors of California prohibited Jean Genet's *The Song of Love* for the overt portrayal of homosexuality in 1966 (ibid, p. 96). With Louis Malle's *The Lovers*, the problem was the description of a housewife's extramarital affair that led British and American censors to ban it from public cinemas (Green & Karolides, 2005, p. 12). Yes, both these countries have boards of film classification still active today, as does Germany, while Australia beat them both for the unofficial title of the most censored country in the "free world"[23] in the 1960s (in Green & Karolides, 2005, p. 140).[24]

Still, no one in the film industry has felt the power of censorship more strongly and comprehensively than Orson Welles. Coming to the business with a superb reputation from the world of theatre and his masterful radio adaptation of *The War of the Worlds*, Welles initially received a uniquely liberal contract for two films, which granted him the right to make all final decisions independently. The first outcome of this was his 1941 *Citizen Kane*, one of the best films in history, still studied and revered today. Aged only twenty-five, Welles, sadly, had already reached the peak of his career. His next film, *The Magnificent Ambersons*, was shortened by producers by forty minutes, despite the contract. The most artistic parts were cut out, and the end was changed to be more optimistic. Welles wrote a fifty-five-page

---

[23] Entries for countries like France, South Africa, Sweden, or Spain in *The Encyclopedia of Censorship* are several pages long and list many examples of censorship not only from the distant past but from our days as well. Those related to Spain, the UK, the US, and the USSR have the length of an essay.

[24] For about four centuries, and until 1968, England had a special censor for theatre, called the Lord Chamberlain or the Master of Revels, which is poignantly portrayed in Tom Stoppard's *Shakespeare in Love*.

long response to the changes, but the producers could not care less (Welles & Bogdanovich, 1998).

To make matters much worse, all of his subsequent projects were barely supported; he had to finance them on his own, or they were shot in Europe.[25] As persona non grata, Welles managed to bring only eight other films (after the *Ambersons*) to full fruition, although his career lasted for more than another four decades. Nevertheless, he remains one of the most influential film directors and actors in history.

Welles was also interrogated during the period of "McCarthyism" when the American senator Joseph McCarthy led anti-communist purges after the end of the Second World War. Although no one admitted it back then, it is now estimated that about 300 film writers, directors, and producers lost their jobs and became proscribed between 1947 and 1957 (Green & Karolides, 2005, p. 576).

The treatment of Orson Welles is only an epitome of the rigid attitude that films should be of standard length and with happy endings to attract larger audiences and earn more money. That is, actually, the way to rank (and ranking would be utterly inapplicable in the wider world of arts) films, film stars, and directors—by calculating the cumulative earnings of their films. Only rare independent films break these patterns and introduce real creativity and imaginativeness in the form of unexpected plot twists and resolutions. Mass media's control of our imagination is so profound and comprehensive that the distinction between pre- and post-television identities was introduced decades ago (Gottschalk, 2000).

Over the last decade, so-called cancel culture became a prominent form of silencing with the advent of social media. It marks a decision of a particular group to boycott altogether (and require that everyone else does the same) a public figure with whose political attitude or form of behaviour they disagree. It all started with the "Me Too" movement but has, in the meantime, spread to issues related to racism, sexism,

---

[25] Welles played in a big-budget propaganda Yugoslavian film about the Second World War (in which Richard Burton played Tito) to earn money for one of his self-financed projects. An urban legend has it that he left a hotel in central Belgrade without paying the bill because he wanted to save as much money as possible. This allegedly helped him finish *Othello*, another of his masterpieces.

ageism, LGBTQI rights, and differences between political parties. That it has promptly grown into a form of silencing was noticed by figures as diverse as Barack Obama, Donald Trump, and Pope Francis II. It has reached the world of (stand-up) comedy as well, the purpose of which is to attack all the limitations imposed on free speech, and some apply it even to the works of artists in whose day and age these notions did not exist, among them Shakespeare, Mozart, and Verdi.

Conclusion

Censorship and silencing have undoubtedly been in operation in all human societies and all historical epochs. Despite their scarcity, creative voices have been regularly exposed to the worst forms of oppression in all too many groups. The more totalitarian the society, the higher the scrutiny of creativity, and it seems that every dictator pays special attention to the control of the arts.

The illustrations of this process offered in this chapter list only a limited number of the most famous cases that took place in the twentieth century. But the censorship of creativity is present today as well, and in all societies, with possible differences in form and degree. Liberties must constantly be won, creative liberties even more than others. Fortunately, there are examples of this as well, to support and embolden future generations of creators.

References

Ardov, M. (2004). *Memories of Shostakovich. Interviews with the Composer's Children*. London: Short Books.

Behrman, S. (2010). *Shostakovich: Socialism, Stalin & Symphonies*. London: Redwords.

Bulgakov, M. (2013). *Diaries and Selected Letters*. London: Alma Classics.

Dimitrijević, A. (2020). Silence and silencing of the traumatised. In: A. Dimitrijević & M. B. Buchholz (Eds.), *Silence and Silencing in Psychoanalysis: Cultural, Clinical and Research Perspectives* (pp. 198–215). London: Routledge.

Dimitrijević, A. (2022). Myth of the solitary artist. In: A. Dimitrijević & M. B. Buchholz (Eds.), *From the Abyss of Loneliness to the Bliss of Solitude* (pp. 103–119). Bicester, UK: Phoenix.

Figes, O. (2007). *Whisperers: Private Life in Stalin's Russia*. London: Penguin.

Finn, P., & Couvée, P. (2014). *The Zhivago affair: The Kremlin, the CIA, and the Battle over a Forbidden Book*. New York: Vintage.

Fulford, K. W. M., Smirnov, A. Y., & Snow, E. (1993). Concepts of disease and the abuse of psychiatry in the USSR. *British Journal of Psychiatry, 162*(6): 801–810.

Gottschalk, S. (2000). Escape from insanity: "Mental disorder" in the post-modern moment. In: D. Fee (Ed.), *Pathology and the Postmodern: Mental Illness as Discourse and Experience* (pp. 18–48). Thousand Oaks, CA: Sage.

Green, J., & Karolides, N. J. (2005). *Encyclopedia of Censorship*. New York: Infobase.

MacDonald, I. (2006). *The New Shostakovich*. London: Pimlico.

Mortimer, L. (2009). *Terror and Joy. The Films of Dušan Makavejev*. Minneapolis, MN: University of Minnesota Press.

Roseberry, E. (1986). *Shostakovich*. London: Omnibus.

Shentalinsky, V. (1996). *Arrested Voices: Resurrecting the Disappeared Writers of the Soviet Regime*. J. Crowfoot (Trans.). New York: The Free Press.

Shostakovich, D. (1981). *Testimony*. S. Volkov (Ed.). London: Faber & Faber.

Tarkovsky, A. (1989). *Sculpting in Time: Reflections on the Cinema*. Austin, TX: University of Texas Press.

True, C. (2002). *American Scream: The Bill Hicks Story*. London: Pan, 2005.

Vučetić, R. (2016). *Monopoly on Truth. Party, Culture, and Censorship in Serbia in the 1960s and 1970s*. Belgrade: Clio. (In Serbian.) Welles, O., & Bogdanovich, P. (1998). *This Is Orson Welles*. New York: Da Capo.

Wilson, E. (2006). *Shostakovich: A Life Remembered*. London: Faber & Faber.

Zappa, F., & Occhiogrosso, P. (1999). *Real Frank Zappa Book*. New York: Simon & Schuster.

CHAPTER 9

Silencing creative voices in the history of psychoanalysis

Aleksandar Dimitrijević

> *There is a great irony at the heart of contemporary psychoanalysis. The skilled psychoanalyst as clinician is, perhaps, the most careful and systematic listener, the most precise and respectful speaker, the most highly trained and refined communicator, that Western culture has produced. A sustained and dedicated effort to discover and articulate the personal meanings, the inner logic of the patient's communications, is the most fundamental dimension of the craft of psychoanalysis in all its variations. Yet, psychoanalysts have enormous difficulty listening and speaking meaningfully to each other.*
>
> (Mitchell, 1991, p. 1)

It is well documented that scientific work and discoveries have often been silenced by ideological or religious institutions and sometimes still are by sources of financial interest. Even in scientific institutions themselves, silencing can occasionally happen due to rivalry, ambition, arrogance, opposition to novelty, or overvaluation of specific ideas or methods. But psychoanalysis is the only discipline that simultaneously aspires to be of a scientific status and establishes its societies and training institutes around the issues of loyalty, dissent, and systematic organised silencing. Not only have the basic concepts been silenced outside the psychoanalytic community, which is still an acute problem in academia, where they are represented in an obsolete and incorrect way or without crediting their origin,[1] but psychoanalysts impede the creative development of their discipline and are most often so used to that impediment that it takes place unrecognised and unopposed (Dimitrijević, 2018, 2019, 2020; Stefana et al., 2021). In this chapter, I will present a historical review of some of the most important cases of silencing creativity in psychoanalytic institutes.

Freud's strategies for silencing

In 1899, Freud, still almost completely unknown to the general public, wrote in *The Interpretation of Dreams* (published the next year) that he had a peculiar problem with maintaining friendships:

> An intimate friend and a hated enemy have always been indispensable requirements for my emotional life; I have always been able to create them anew, and not infrequently my childish ideal has been so closely approached that friend and enemy coincided in the same person. (1900a, p. 385)

By that point, this dynamic was evident in Freud's relationships with Joseph Breuer and Wilhelm Fliess. Both were close friends and essential sources of intellectual and financial support, with whom Freud exchanged many new ideas in frequent conversations and correspondence. Breuer mentored Freud, referred patients to him, and gave him money. But as soon as Breuer or Fliess started developing their ideas or showed a lack of missionary zeal for Freud's theory, when, in other words, Freud thought they would not contribute to his limitless ambitions (see Breger, 2009), he terminated contacts and treated them

---

[1] Gail Hornstein (1992) has reviewed numerous psychology textbooks and noticed that "textbook writers took advantage of their role by assimilating psychoanalytic concepts into mainstream psychology without mentioning their origins" (p. 260). For more recent reviews, see Habarth et al., 2011; Park, 2006.

almost as enemies. It was enough for Breuer to say one sentence about his disagreement with Freud's conviction that all hysterical symptoms are related to sexuality, after he had been the only colleague who publicly defended Freud.[2] In every subsequent iteration of the treatment of Anna O., Breuer would turn into a more and more incompetent and unreliable character: Freud's famous 1909 Clark lectures open with giving Breuer due credit for the invention of psychoanalysis, but his correspondence of 1932 makes a caricature of the whole history, which was again exaggerated even further in Jones's biography of Freud (see Breger, 2000, pp. 122–124). When they met in the street many years after the end of their friendship and collaboration, Freud refused to greet Breuer (Breger, 2000, p. 125), which is another pattern that will be repeated.

The next examples followed almost immediately. In 1902, Freud founded the "Wednesday Society", which would transform into the Vienna Psychoanalytic Society on April 15, 1907. But, as he would later write in his *An Autobiographical Study*, "For more than ten years after my separation from Breuer I had no followers" (1925d, p. 48). He was never satisfied with friends or collaborators, not even with associates or assistants. The expression "my followers"[3] can easily have a religious connotation (devotee, believer), and Freud had started using it much earlier.[4] Freud wrote to Fliess on December 14, 1899, almost immediately after *The Interpretation of Dreams* was published: "Your news of the dozen readers in Berlin pleases me greatly. I must have some readers here as well; the time is not yet ripe for followers." The word "follower" then appears quite regularly in his correspondence with Jung, public lectures (1916–1917), and his accounts of psychoanalytic

---

[2] Biographers also hypothesise that Freud wanted to get away from his dependence on Breuer and establish relationships with colleagues where he would be the dominant figure (see Breger, 2000, ch. 7; Breger, 2009; Grosskurth, 1991, p. 7).

[3] In Freud's letter to Fliess of December 14, 1899, he uses the term "Anhängerschaft". "Anhänger" is used in German to define a group of religious or political companions who believe they share privileged abilities or knowledge, considered "exclusive". The distinction of inside ("belongs to us") vs outside ("does not belong to us") is inherent in this terminology.

[4] And when Freud used the word "students" (Schülern), like in *The Psychopathology of Everyday Life* ("the circle of my students"—1901b, p. 150), the English translation uses "followers", which was a custom by the 1920s.

history—"Five Lectures on Psycho-Analysis" (1910a), "On the History of the Psycho-Analytic Movement" (1914d), and *An Autobiographical Study* (1925d). And when we study various sources, and not just the Freud–Jones version of the history of psychoanalysis, we can easily see that it is precisely *followers* he was looking for and that there was nothing more important for any member of the movement than to be a loyal follower.

Wilhelm Stekel and Alfred Adler were among the first members of the Wednesday Society and the earliest supporters and propagators of psychoanalysis. But two crucial things had changed by March 1910, the time of the Nuremberg Psychoanalytic Congress. First of all, there was a large group of followers who were fighting for the attention of the leader, many of whom were in bitter rivalry against those who had recognised him earlier on. To make matters worse, both Stekel and Adler had been developing in their own ways, trying to provide creative additions and amendments to Freud's theories. But they were soon to learn that this was not allowed. While in the words of one former IPA president, "[Freud] welcomed contributions from his adherents so long as they were fully compatible with his positions, and usually, just extensions or amplifications of them" (Wallerstein, 2004, p. 201), those who did not follow his doctrine were soon ostracised without any hope of redemption. To use the case of Stekel as an illustration, as soon as he wrote a book Freud inspected and did not entirely approve of, the relationship had to be terminated, although Stekel was the vice president of the Vienna Psychoanalytic Society.[5] Not only had all loyal followers stopped quoting Stekel and started writing papers against him, but Freud was angry at Stekel until the end of his life, never replied to his friendly and caring letters, and in his correspondences called him a "swine" and a "terrible man" (Rudnytsky, 2011).

As an essential tool for both the propagation and control of psychoanalysis, the early journals were founded already before the First World War. The first one was *The Annual of Psychoanalysis*, and Freud asked to have the power of veto against any submitted paper he did not want to see published (Grosskurth, 1991, p. 10). However, the editor-in-chief was

---

[5] To make things even more ironic, the president was Adler. They both resigned after only four months in the office.

Stekel, and he refused to renounce the position after leaving the society. Freud thus initiated two other journals and installed more trusted people as editors: *Imago*, with Rank and Sachs, and *The International Journal of Medical Psychoanalysis*, with Jones, Ferenczi, and Rank.

Sándor Ferenczi met Freud in 1908 and almost immediately became a most zealous supporter, idealising Freud's personality and theory to the extreme (Dimitrijević et al., 2018). Because of his wish to protect Freud's sexual drive doctrine from any heresies, he suggested founding an international society of Freud's followers. The primary purpose of this group, inaugurated at the Nuremberg Congress and named the International Psychoanalytical Association, was to defend Freud's theory from external criticisms and prohibit people from calling themselves psychoanalysts without Freud's permission, or as he called them "wild analysts" (Freud, 1910k).

Whoever labelled psychoanalysis a Jewish science did it for the wrong reason. Its problems were not related to its members belonging to the same cultural background; it is that it was organised as a quasi-religious sect. Some participants recognised this early. This is how the musicologist Max Graf, father of "Little Hans", described the beginnings:

> There was an atmosphere of the foundation of a religion in that room. Freud himself was its new prophet who made the theretofore prevailing methods of psychological investigation appear superficial. Freud's pupils—all inspired and convinced—were his apostles. (Quoted in Rudnytsky, 2002, p. 200)

The first president of the IPA was Carl Gustav Jung. When elected in 1910, he was still a loyal and fervent Freudian. The correspondence between the two men is full of religious metaphors of the weirdest kind. For instance, Freud wrote to Jung on January 17, 1909: "If I am Moses, then you are the Joshua and will take possession of the promised land of psychiatry." Even as late as 1925, Freud wrote in his *Autobiographical Study* (referring to Jung) that "A 'Christ' had to stand at the forefront of the movement" (p. 556). Freud was initially fascinated by Jung and chose him as the "heir to the throne" because Jung was almost the only gentile in the group. They spoke for hours on end, sometimes eight, once thirteen; exchanged hundreds of letters; travelled together and visited each other's families. The end started when Freud required Jung to defend the "fortress of libido theory", and it turned out that Jung saw libido as "l'élan vital" (and not exclusively sexual energy) and was a different kind of a believer. Mutual accusations led to Jung's resignation, then total distance, and finally to the foundation of another quasi-religious group organised almost in the same way as the initial one. But sadly, it did not end there. Freud recruited Ferenczi to write against Jung (letter of October 20, 1913), in ways from a savagely critical review of one of his books (Ferenczi, 1913) to propagandistic letters. And the spite never went away, as we can learn from an interview Henry A. Murray gave to James Anderson about his meeting with Freud over Christmas week in 1937:

> ... that was interesting because [Freud] wanted to see me, I found out. Of course, I went there to see him. But before I had a chance to put in my oar, I got an invitation to see him, and I couldn't make out what this was. I didn't see any sense in it until I got there and then he said right away, "Why didn't I get an honorary degree at the Harvard Tercentenary and Jung got one?" (Anderson, 2017, p. 323)

Almost twenty-five years later, at the age of eighty-one, Freud still collected information about Jung and was passionate about having at least equal appreciation!

In 1914, Freud wrote a brief text about the history of psychoanalysis (1914d). This sounds surprising as only twenty years had passed since the publication of *Studies on Hysteria*. However, the true purpose becomes evident when we remember that it was written immediately after the early "dissidents" were out and with the basic idea of setting clear boundaries against the approaches of Adler and Jung. Another detail that stands out as very illuminating is in the very title, "On the History of the Psycho-analytic Movement". Freud named psychoanalysis a "movement" as if it belonged in the political or religious domains, although he insisted it was a scientific discipline.

And indeed, the Jung crisis made Freud, if anything, more rigid and authoritarian. He did not revise or even test a single detail of his theories, but at Ernest Jones's suggestion, he formed a secret body focused on preventing future "heresies" and protecting the purity of his quasi-religion. It was Ferenczi's idea that "a small group of colleagues could be analysed by Freud so that they could represent the pure theory unadulterated by personal complexes, and thus build an official inner circle in the Association" (Jones to Freud, July 30, 1912). It turned out that Freud had already had such an idea: "I hoped Jung would collect such a circle around him … it would make my living and dying easier for me if I knew of such an association existing to watch over my creation" (Freud to Jones, August 1, 1912).[6]

The so-called "Secret Committee" consisted of seven members: Freud himself, Karl Abraham, Max Eitingon,[7] Sándor Ferenczi, Ernest Jones, Otto Rank, and Hans Sachs. Over more than ten years, they exchanged hundreds of letters (from 1920 onward circular letters), met many times, led heated debates, and plotted against other people and one another. The Committee was a body as ideological as there ever was one. The members were bound by wearing the same rings with the figure of Oedipus, a present from Freud to all others; they read and approved each submitted manuscript and made significant organisational and political decisions. All presidents of the IPA and the editors of *The International Journal of Psychoanalysis* came from inside this group for almost half a century. Freud insisted on absolute secrecy (letter to Jones, August 1, 1912), and it was only with the publication of significant books of "circular letters" and correspondence between Freud and the individual Committee members, which started in the 1980s, that we became aware of its existence and came to understand that the Committee's primary purpose was to silence every unorthodox (deviant) opinion and organise the psychoanalytic community based on the principles of loyalty and obedience (Wittenberger, 1988).

Freud kept all the Committee members dependent on him for all these years and referred to them as his "adopted children".

---

[6] In a curious example of silencing, Jones, in his *Biography*, omitted these sentences, although the rest of that letter was quoted (Grosskurth, 1991, p. 47). It is difficult to ascertain the reason, but one can speculate that Jones either did not want the reader to see that the originator of the idea was Freud and not Ferenczi or that even he found Freud's constant mention of dying too melodramatic.

[7] Eitingon only joined in 1919.

His "fatherly role" was mentioned to Ferenczi in 1931, when Ferenczi was fifty-seven years old (letter of December 13). Freud briefly analysed Ferenczi in 1914–1916 (see Bonomi, 2018), paid for Rank's studies, and analysed Jones's wife, Loe Kann. He never stopped analysing all of them in meetings and correspondences. They analysed the former members constantly, believing that the reason for "heresy" had to be a mental disorder. At the same moment, Freud himself was unanalysed, never supervised, and never found any responsibility in his attitudes or behaviour. As Jung was announcing his distance and resignation, Freud recognised that he felt about himself that "there is some piece of unruly homosexual feeling at the root of the matter" (letter to Jones of December 8, 1912). Yet this was never communicated openly to Jung, analysis or supervision was not sought, and all the blame was put on Jung.

The Committee members were in almost constant rivalrous battles. For instance, Jones described that Rank was "somewhat deteriorating" and that his way of "conducting business was distinctly Oriental" (letter to A. A. Brill of April 9, 1923, quoted in Grosskurth, 1991, p. 133). Ferenczi learned about this from Brill, but now (most probably in Ferenczi's mind), the anti-Semitic remark "distinctly Oriental" turned into "a swindling Jew". Ferenczi shared with all the other members what he believed Jones had written, so Rank demanded that Jones be expelled from the Committee.

Ironically, some Committee members experienced the same destiny they had previously prepared for others. By the mid-1920s, no psychoanalytic institute allowed reading or even mentioning Adler or Jung, while, at the same moment, Rank was the editor of journals and the publishing house, as well as Freud's former personal secretary.[8] In the fateful period of 1923–1924, Sándor Ferenczi and Otto Rank proposed, in their joint book *Development of Psychoanalysis*,[9] that instead of metapsychology, we should use the analytic situation as a defining feature of psychoanalysis. All this was in part a reaction to Freud's

---

[8] Freud trusted Rank so much that Rank authored two chapters that were included in some editions of *The Interpretation of Dreams*. They were, of course, excluded after the conflict.

[9] The actual title of the book should have been translated as "The Developmental Aims of Psychoanalysis".

introduction of the "death drive" since the authors believed that he had paid far more attention to abstract concepts than to issues of clinical technique: "Psychoanalytic method had fossilized, [Ferenczi] believed, and become an overly intellectualized process of educating patients about the contents of their unconscious" (Makari, 2008, p. 352; see also Kirsch et al., 2022). The invitation to focus on transference, resistance, and the actual analytic relationship was seen as too revolutionary for the mid-1920s and led to Freud's dismissal of the two men he had considered worthy of being his heir.[10] Today, this attitude is being taken for granted, so much so that it is difficult to believe that psychoanalysts have ever worked in a different way.

Rank's "Trauma of Birth" (1924) was initially praised by Freud as the most original psychoanalytic publication ever, only to become so unacceptable for Freud that he wrote a whole paper against it (*Inhibitions, Symptoms and Anxiety* (1926d)) and induced others into doing the same. One blatant example is that Ferenczi refused to greet Rank, his long-term friend, when they met in New York City in 1927 (see Falzeder, 2015). Then, of course, Rank immediately disappeared from psychoanalytic journals, curricula, or conferences, although he kept exerting a significant influence on the field of social work, on the use of and research on empathy, on Carl Rogers, but never again on mainstream psychoanalysis (Janus, 2010, 2014; Winthuis, 2006). To make matters additionally bizarre, Rank was replaced on the Committee by Anna Freud, the daughter Freud had secretly analysed himself.

And what Ferenczi did to Rank (and Jung before that) struck him as a massive injustice when it happened to him several years later. When he tried to develop the psychoanalytic technique for work with severely traumatised patients, Freud accused him of much more than he had ever done,[11] and when Ferenczi wrote about the importance and high frequency of actual trauma (Ferenczi, 1949), Freud, predictably, ceased contact with him and wrote to other people about him in derogatory ways. Six days after Ferenczi's death, Freud wrote to Jones: "… for years Ferenczi has no longer been with us, indeed, not even with himself. It is

---

[10] Less importantly, Freud had also wanted Ferenczi to marry his daughter Mathilde and become his son-in-law.
[11] See the letter of December 13 1931.

now easier to comprehend the slow process of destruction to which he fell victim ... a mental degeneration in the form of paranoia developed with uncanny logical consistency ... in this confusion his once brilliant intelligence was extinguished" (letter of May 29, 1933). The silencing of Ferenczi's final and groundbreaking papers lasted for more than half a century, until Judith Dupont managed to publish his diary in French and English (see Dimitrijević, 2021, 2022).

In 1917, Freud received a letter from Georg Groddeck, a German physician many now consider the father of psychosomatics (for details, see Dimitrijević, 2008). Groddeck joined the movement, and Freud took the term "das Es" from him (translated into English as "the It" in the context of Groddeck's theory and "the Id" in Freud's). Groddeck remained Sándor Ferenczi's lifelong friend, but he described himself as "the wild analyst" and, over time, distanced himself from Freud and many other analysts, disappointed by their dogmatism.

In all of these cases, it is only the details that have slightly changed, while the basic pattern has, every time, remained entirely the same. Freud does not seem to have even considered the possibility of him being at fault and, at the same time, initiated the silencing and dismissal of all criticisms of psychoanalysis with the use of ad hominem argumentation focused on the alleged mental disorder in his former friends/ analysands and now enemies. The explanations followed a well-known pattern: unresolved father complex, repressed homicidality, paranoia, delusions, and jealousy (Bergmann, 2004; see also Dimitrijević, 2007a). In his eyes, Freud was always a completely innocent victim. Additional reasons were offered with the hope that they could explain what was named the "problem of dissidence" in psychoanalysis (Bergmann, 2004): resistance towards Freud's personality; basic attitude of ingratitude and criticism; unsuccessful training analyses; structural flaws in the organisation of training institutes—this one most persistently by a former president of the IPA (Kernberg, 1986, 1992, 1996, 2000, 2012; see also Buchholz & Dimitrijević, 2018; Dimitrijević, 2018); requirement of conviction in the postulates of psychoanalysis—and convictions can be gained and lost; the vague idea of what constitutes progress in psychoanalysis and how it can be verified (Stepansky, 2009).

The abuse of psychoanalytic concepts to silence critics, all based on the quasi-religious belief that these concepts were perfect as they were and could not be improved without Freud's blessing, remained in use by other psychoanalysts even long after Freud's death. This should not surprise us, as the selection process was biased, with loyalty much preferred to creativity, so decision-makers could not have been much different in the coming generations.

Post-Freudian psychoanalytic censorship

While Freud was still alive, Wilhelm Reich was expelled by virtually every group he belonged to (Nitzschke, 1992; Peglau, 2013; Rubin, 2002; Zweig, 1971). A wunderkind of sorts, Reich taught psychoanalytic technique while still in his twenties and in Vienna. Yet he was seen as too political. He joined the Communist International and advocated that economic liberation was only half the way and that sexual liberation was also necessary. That led to him being expelled from the German Psychoanalytic Society and subsequently from the Danish and Norwegian ones (where he lived between 1934 and 1939). On what grounds, one might wonder, but there is no clear solution to that puzzle apart from the standard—he was not an orthodox, obedient believer. That he would later die in a prison cell after his books were burned in the US in 1955 makes his case even more relevant and tragic.

The effort to secure that all the psychoanalysts would speak unisono continued after Freud's death, with the only major novelty that there were now several sources of authority instead of only one. This made it evident that "dissidence" resulted from the lack of open exchange of opinions, which, as usual in scientific communities, can and should be controversial until a mode of resolving controversies is established. Alas, "psychoanalysis is the only science without data, and the only hermeneutics without a text" (Siegel et al., 2002, p. 410).

Melanie Klein worked hard on establishing a group of "Kleinian analysts". Her efforts included scheming and influencing even her then-current analysands, like Paula Heimann, to vote in her favour and actively silencing authors who pursued their creativity, like Donald Winnicott and John Bowlby.

Heimann, known to us as the theorist of countertransference, was born as a "replacement child" after the death of a sister and entered analysis with Klein after she had consoled Klein over the death of one of her sons, and become to Klein a kind of replacement for her estranged daughter Melitta Schmideberg. No wonder she wanted to say something about countertransference. Very specific silencing happened later on, and, in the words of Franco Borgogno (2007, p. 65), Heimann could remember

> the pain, the malaise, the anger and the conflict she experienced at not being able to speak her mind and having to limit herself to carrying out orders, once she had been invited into the circle of the "great" to write papers supporting Klein; at the same time, she could not even openly declare that she was still in analysis with her, since she was the "heiress to the throne" and if she had done so, she would have compromised the "queen" before the society.

The story is completely the same as with Freud and members of his secret committee: silencing, secrets, intrigue, abusing the powers of the analyst, thrones, including disrespect of the analyst–patient boundaries.

Winnicott was among the first five "Kleinian analysts" in London. He had a strong wish to be analysed by Klein but, at her insistence, analysed one of her sons. Winnicott somehow managed to resist Klein's pressure to let her supervise his analysis of her son. Yet, after his 1952 presentation of what was later to be published as "Transitional Objects and Transitional Phenomena", she never replied to his letters again, even when he explicitly asked her to support his creativity. On the surface, she could not care less, but the two might have been in a silent dialogue through seemingly independent papers on the same topics (see Caldwell, 2022).

Even worse with John Bowlby, Klein's one-time supervisee, who always emphasised the importance of actual interpersonal relationships and not only mental objects.[12] This deviation from Klein's model got Bowlby entirely ostracised from the psychoanalytic community—in the words of Jeremy Holmes (1993, p. 4), "as a dissident in Stalin's Soviet Union"—and he was forced to publish elsewhere until the end of his life, to be rediscovered by psychoanalysts only afterwards.

---

[12] Bowlby, allegedly, at a meeting of the British Psychoanalytical Society, in 1955, jumped to his feet and very loudly said, "But bad mothers do exist!"

This same attitude was expressed as recently as 2006 when Hanna Segal claimed that the Freud–Klein–Bion[13] model is a search for truth, while the Independents (specifically: Ferenczi, Balint, Winnicott, and Kohut) "invite the patient to live in a lie" (p. 289).

Anna Freud, on the other hand, was never much focused on building her cult and followers. Instead, she aimed more than anything else at preserving the idealised image of her father as a person and psychoanalyst. To ensure this, she did not allow the publication of any of his preserved correspondences; indeed, only the letters he exchanged with Jung were available uncensored before she died in 1982.[14] This is usually understood as a daughter's loyalty to her father, while one cannot but wonder whether it comes from the former analysand's idealisations that were never completely worked through.

A fitting illustration of Anna Freud's efforts at silencing is her letter to Michael Balint of June 3, 1952, in which she demanded of him not to share parts of Freud–Ferenczi correspondence with Ernest Jones, who was working on his Freud biography:

> Recently, I have been involved with Jones in various regards because of my father's biography and after some consideration, we have handed Jones the letters my parents wrote to one another during their years of engagement, which, so far, no one had read before us, for review. The work Jones is doing on the biography is very impressive. I have read the first chapters and I admire his objective, factual and scientific attitude towards the whole subject matter.
>
> Under this impression, I am starting to doubt, after all, whether we are doing right by withholding Ferenczi's letters from him. Should we change our minds? If so, it would have to be reviewed whether letters include personal remarks about Jones himself, because these must surely not be given to him.

---

[13] To the best of my knowledge, it remains open for future study to establish whether there is a contextual reason for the blossoming of Wilfred Bion's creativity only after the death of Melanie Klein and his moving out of London.

[14] A selection of Freud's letters was edited by his son Ernst (1960), as well as a part of the correspondence with Fliess that was considered "safe".

What do you think?[15]

Anna Freud here admits her suspicions about Jones and her withdrawing some historical materials from him, all with the purpose, initially, of controlling what would appear in his Freud biography, and now of protecting him from discovering Freud's genuine opinion about Jones. In the 1950s, the practices of withdrawing, censoring, selection, and silencing are still actively in use.

The distrust Anna Freud felt towards Jones, whom she had known since childhood, stems from a problem that only a limited number of persons were aware of at that time. Jones had been taken to court on the charge of sexual molestation based on independent testimonies of several schoolgirls in London at the beginning of the century and then in Canada in 1912. The archival work of Philip Kuhn (2002a, 2002b, 2014a, 2014b, 2015) very strongly suggests that Jones did commit these crimes. Kuhn had discovered a police record about one set of medical examinations Jones performed, which said that "the stains (on the tablecloth) were of such a character that they should not have been there" and claimed that no other interpretation of the "stains" is possible but that they were traces of semen (2002a, p. 397). Correspondences show that Ferenczi, as Jones's analyst, Freud, and Jung were aware of this. When the eighteen-year-old Anna Freud was alone in England in 1914, Freud used two long letters to warn her about the danger of Jones's "serious intentions of wooing you" (July 16, 1914). He shared what he had learned analysing Jones's first wife and warned Anna that "Dr Jones needs a wife to protect him from the temptations that a doctor is exposed to" (July 22, 1914). No similar kind of protection was offered to Jones's patients, analysands, supervisees, and colleagues when he was being promoted to all the positions of power in psychoanalytic institutions.

Jones himself was one of the highest censors of British psychoanalysis. Both president of the IPA and editor of *The International Journal of Psychoanalysis* for almost twenty-five years (1932–1955), he made many fateful decisions, the most interesting of which are related to Sándor Ferenczi, his former analyst. Throughout the 1950s, Jones opposed

---

[15] This unpublished letter is today at the Balint Archive at the University of Essex. It was kindly translated by Alma Schlegel, MA.

Balint's efforts to publish Ferenczi's legacy (the last four papers,[16] for which he was excommunicated, correspondence with Freud, and the *Clinical Diary*), portrayed Ferenczi as psychotic in the third volume of his biography of Freud (1957) and tried to silence Balint and other colleagues who were first-hand witnesses of Ferenczi's final illness. When Ferenczi's *Diary* was finally published by Judith Dupont in 1985 in French and 1988 in English, more than half a century after his death, no one wrote of it as a product of madness (Dimitrijević, 2022), but it was experienced as an earthquake that led to the so-called Ferenczi renaissance (Dimitrijević, 2021).

On the other side of the ocean, the American Psychoanalytic Association was probably even more conservative. As a result, many of the most creative authors and liberal-minded institutes were never accepted into APsaA, like the Chestnut Lodge Hospital (Frieda Fromm-Reichmann, Harold Searles), Washington Psychoanalytic Society (Harry Stack Sullivan, Clara Thompson), William Alanson White Institute (Karen Hornay, Erich Fromm, Edgar Levenson, Steven Mitchell, Jay Greenberg). What made them ineligible for membership in APsaA was their interpersonal approach, focusing on the analytic relationship rather than on the setting, especially in their work with psychotic patients (Hornstein, 2000; see also Dimitrijević, 2007b). For example, at one conference, Frieda Fromm-Reichmann was asked by an enraged Edward Bibring, "What right do you have to call yourself a psychoanalyst?" (see Silver, 2018, pp. 217ff.). Not surprisingly, the person who expressed that judgement hidden within a question (see Blass, 2010) has not made a single creative contribution to psychoanalysis.

Almost immediately after the Second World War, Kurt Eissler started interviewing anyone who had any contact with Freud and assembling historical documents related to him. He founded The Sigmund Freud Archives, now housed by the Library of Congress in Washington, DC. Unlike archives that researchers can use, however, this is a massive collection of documents, most of which were classified, and Eissler held

---

[16] Given that these papers emphasise the detrimental effects of early childhood neglect and abuse, the aforementioned biographical details might offer an explanation as to why Jones did not want them published and discussed.

the keys to the "forbidden knowledge" he—and Anna Freud—would grant only to the chosen few. The proportions of this fight for control and silencing began to become evident during the 1980s after Eissler had selected Jeffrey Masson to be the archive director, and Masson published the complete Freud–Fliess correspondence (1985) and exposed the whole enterprise. Masson was speedily fired; he moved to New Zealand and severed all ties with the psychoanalytic community, while the Archives were digitised in 2017, yet its large parts remain classified, and some will not become open for a couple more decades. It is impossible to reconcile this secretiveness with the spirits of psychoanalysis focused on personal honesty and disclosure and of science focused on exploring everything there is.

One of the most impressive stories of integrity in the face of psychoanalytic authoritarianism is that of Erich Fromm (for details, see Rudnytsky, 2019). Profoundly influenced by the independent spirits of Frieda Fromm-Reichmann, his first wife, and both Groddeck and Ferenczi, Fromm openly criticised the psychoanalytic establishment as early as 1935. Over time, Fromm was ostracised by both the IPA (in 1953) and the Frankfurt "Institute for Social Research" and developed his original ideas in publications that sold millions of copies in countless translations. In 1959, Fromm was the first to expose the methods of "Stalinist history" after Jones had described Rank and Ferenczi as psychotic. That same year, Fromm published a book that analysed Freud's authoritarianism (*The Mission of Sigmund Freud*).

In 1957, Heinz Kohut's plenary address at the APsaA annual meeting was so severely criticised by all four discussants that he hardly published anything in the following years. His sin? He advocated the inevitability of empathy, nowadays accepted by almost everyone but unacceptable in the era of rigid adherence to the idea of the analyst as neutral, abstinent, and anonymous. As a result, the paper based on the presentation (Kohut, 1959) was rejected by several psychoanalytic journals and published only after the intervention of one influential member (Maxwell Gitelson), unrelated to scientific discussion or arguments. This certainly contributed to the decision by the former "Mr Psychoanalysis" to establish a new school outside of APsaA. The degree of Kohut's traumatisation from this attempt at unsilencing is also evident from the fact that his last two papers (1981, 1982) were both focused on empathy, and both mention the 1957 panel.

If this overview seems like it refers to the events from the distant past, the case Carlo Bonomi describes in the first volume of his *The Cut and the Building of Psychoanalysis* (2015) shows that the same trends are still active today, in *The International Journal of Psychoanalysis*, the allegedly most important, or at least most widely read publication. Bonomi submitted a paper about female castration as a medical procedure in the nineteenth century and its influence on Freud and the foundation of psychoanalysis. His "endless and continuing odyssey" (Bonomi, 2015, p. 7) started with the support and advice of the editor that the paper was rich and should be divided into two parts. But when the first part was submitted, "a member of the editorial board objected to my thesis and vetoed the publication" (ibid.). Although it may be hard to believe, the right to veto a paper, and not reject it based on problems with relevance, methodology, and conclusion, as expected in the scientific community, existed as recently as 2007 or 2008!? The paper was finally published (Bonomi, 2009), but only after the journal had changed its rules and after a year-long conflict inside the editorial board. Unfortunately, the next episode did not reach such a favourable resolution, as the second part of the paper was rejected, even though it was the editor's idea to divide the initial manuscript. It was, however, accepted by *Psychoanalytic Quarterly* and published in 2013. Carlo Bonomi confessed: "I still don't know why the psychoanalytic community had to be protected from a simple paper which treated the history of the castration of women by male doctors" (2015, p. 9).

I find this question extremely relevant. Why, indeed, does anyone believe that the psychoanalytic community or theories need protection? And from its members? Also: who has the mandate to decide on this, and how have they obtained it? The only answer I can come up with is that what is being protected here is the traumatising order of Freud's strictly hierarchical, quasi-religious group of adoring, obedient, loyal, adopted sons, which still survives and flourishes today.

Silencing, brain drain, and the founders of other psychotherapy schools

In a rare book focused on the issue of dissidence in psychoanalysis, the renowned New York based psychoanalyst and author Martin Bergmann claimed that

> Freud not only created psychoanalysis but during his lifetime no psychoanalyst but Freud wrote papers that have survived as milestones in the history of psychoanalysis ... During Freud's lifetime, he was psychoanalysis. He was the father but also almost the only creator of psychoanalysis. To disagree with Freud was for psychoanalysts as well as dissidents, an act of patricide. (2004, p. 261)

The personal opinion Bergmann wants to present as a fact is, in my view, easily disputable, given the contributions of Ferenczi, Rank, Abraham, Klein, Groddeck, and many others. The conclusion is, however, successfully imposed by Freud on his early followers and then by them on the subsequent generations of psychoanalysts. We are taught to see only Freud and forget about anyone else's originality. I want to concentrate on the consequences of this situation, which remain insufficiently explored.

Few communities have suffered from such a debilitating brain drain as the psychoanalytic one has for more than a century. Starting with Adler and Jung, a host of creative persons, be they members or candidates or supporters, have left and developed different, often related and relevant ideas, which they were not allowed to discuss with their fellow psychoanalysts. In several cases, they founded psychology and psychotherapy schools, some considered contradictory and rivalrous to psychoanalysis.

It is, of course, well known that Adlerian and Jungian institutes exist throughout Europe and the US, as well as in Japan, yet dialogue with them is still scarce. Therefore, it is mere speculation to wonder whether Adler is completely absorbed within the theory of narcissism and power and whether Jung had a direct influence on post-Kleinian approaches that have developed the idea of preconceptions, as we know so little about each other. Moreover, Lacanian theory is increasingly influential in philosophy and humanities, but establishing a dialogue seems even more complicated there.

Humanistic psychology, once "the third force in psychology", regularly seen as the opposite of psychoanalysis, was founded by former psychoanalysts. Abraham Maslow was a trained psychoanalyst; Carl Rogers was analysed by Otto Rank; and Erich Fromm was not only an essential author but also an early challenger of psychoanalytic dogmas.

However, when they discovered psychoanalysis was too constrained for all of their interests and concerns, they had to leave, as the option of broadening psychoanalytic horizons did not exist.

Worse still, Aaron Beck's promotion was slowed down even though he had graduated from the Philadelphia Psychoanalytic Institute, probably because he advocated the importance of empirical research in psychoanalysis. Beck left APsaA and founded cognitive behavioural therapy, which has overpowered psychoanalysis in most Western countries, and psychoanalysts are nowadays more aware of the importance of empirical research.[17]

Alexander Lowen, the founder of bioenergetics, was analysed by Wilhelm Reich, while the Gestalt therapist Fritz Perls and the transactional analyst Eric Berne started as psychoanalysts, all of them writing variations of psychoanalytic ideas alongside original ideas and techniques, which psychoanalysis has not benefitted from as we have differentiated from them and often hold them in contempt. And who could count the number of people who contributed to these other approaches developing their founders' ideas and could have enriched psychoanalysis?

Conclusion

Although psychoanalysts, in their clinical work, aim at enabling people to voice their unexpressed and often silenced pains (Dimitrijević, 2020; Dimitrijević & Buchholz, 2020), it seems apparent that they often do the opposite to one another. Since their establishment, psychoanalytic institutions have controlled, suppressed, censored, and ostracised many of their members. Putting loyalty and the idolisation of Freud before any other values, they have thwarted creativity and jeopardised the future of the whole discipline. Freud himself laid the foundations for this, and sadly, many influential figures in the coming and current generations applied the same ideological and quasi-religious approach.

Because of this, any activity that is not a repetition is discouraged by rules, written and unwritten, and communication, explicit and silent.

---

[17] The number of psychoanalysts who perform empirical research is still tiny compared to the total number of authors or publications (Stefana et al., 2021).

Where innovation leads to being excluded and attacked, people do not freely associate, explore, wonder, question, challenge, learn from other disciplines and sciences … Curiosity is anaesthetised when the boundaries of thinking are already set, and everyone knows about the punishment prepared for those who dare go beyond. Given the dire position of psychoanalysis in the contemporary world, its destiny might depend precisely on this—breaking the history and patterns of silencing in psychoanalytic institutions and developing the spirit of free exchange and innovation.

References

Anderson, J. W. (2017). An interview with Henry A. Murray on his meeting with Sigmund Freud. *Psychoanalytic Psychology, 34*(3): 322–331.

Bergmann, M. S. (2004). Rethinking dissidence and change in the history of psychoanalysis. In: M. S. Bergmann (Ed.), *Understanding Dissidence and Controversy in the History of Psychoanalysis* (pp. 1–109). New York: Other Press.

Blass, R. B. (2010). Affirming "That's not psycho-analysis!" On the value of the politically incorrect act of attempting to define the limits of our field. *International Journal of Psychoanalysis, 91*: 81–99.

Bonomi, C. (2009). The relevance of castration and circumcision to the origins of psychoanalysis: 1. The medical context. *International Journal of Psychoanalysis, 90*(3): 551–580.

Bonomi, C. (2013). Withstanding trauma: The significance of Emma Eckstein's circumcision to Freud's Irma dream. *Psychoanalytic Quarterly, 82*(3): 689–740.

Bonomi, C. (2015). *The Cut and the Building of Psychoanalysis, Volume I: Sigmund Freud and Emma Eckstein.* London: Routledge.

Bonomi, C. (2018). Ferenczi's analyses with Freud. In: A. Dimitrijevic, G. Cassullo, & J. B. Frankel (Eds.), *Ferenczi's Influence on Contemporary Psychoanalytic Traditions* (pp. 30–37). London: Routledge.

Borgogno, F. P. (2007). *Psychoanalysis as a Journey.* London: Open Gate.

Breger, L. (2000). *Freud: Darkness in the Midst of Vision.* Hoboken, NJ: John Wiley & Sons.

Breger, L. (2009). *A Dream of Undying Fame: How Freud Betrayed His Mentor and Invented Psychoanalysis.* New York: Basic Books.

Buchholz, M. B., & Dimitrijević, A. (2018). Editorial: Teaching for survival. *International Forum of Psychoanalysis*, *27*(2): 73–75.

Caldwell, L. (2022). Loneliness and being alone: the contributions of two British analysts. In: A. Dimitrijević & M. B. Buchholz (Eds.), *From the Abyss of Loneliness to the Bliss of Solitude: Cultural, Social and Psychoanalytic Perspectives* (pp. 267–277). Bicester, UK: Phoenix.

Dimitrijević, A. (2007a). "Understanding Dissidence and Controversy in the History of Psychoanalysis" edited by Martin S. Bergmann. *International Forum of Psychoanalysis*, *16*(1): 55–59.

Dimitrijević, A. (2007b). "To Redeem One Person Is to Redeem the World. The Life of Frieda Fromm-Reichmann" by Gail A. Hornstein. *International Forum of Psychoanalysis*, *16*(2): 132–134.

Dimitrijević, A. (2008). Definition, foundation, and the meaning of illness: Locating Georg Groddeck in the history of medicine. *American Journal of Psychoanalysis*, *68*(2): 139–147.

Dimitrijević, A. (2018). A mixed model for psychoanalytic education. *International Forum of Psychoanalysis*, *27*(2): 121–125.

Dimitrijević, A. (2019). Is integration possible for psychoanalysis? In: A. Borgos, F. Eros, & J. Gyimesi (Eds.), *Psychology and Politics* (pp. 345–352). Budapest: Central European University.

Dimitrijević, A. (2020). Silence and silencing of the traumatised. In: A. Dimitrijević & M. B. Buchholz (Eds.), *Silence and Silencing in Psychoanalysis: Cultural, Clinical and Research Perspectives* (pp. 198–215). London: Routledge.

Dimitrijević, A. (2021). "As Time Goes By: An Analytic Journey" by Judith Dupont. *American Journal of Psychoanalysis*, *81*(2): 263–267.

Dimitrijević, A. (2022). "Born in the middle of psychoanalysis". An interview with Judith Dupont. *American Journal of Psychoanalysis*, *82*(4): 548–573. https://doi.org/10.1057/s11231-022-09372-9.

Dimitrijević, A., & Buchholz, M. B. (Eds.) (2020). *Silence and Silencing in Psychoanalysis: Cultural, Clinical and Research Perspectives*. London: Routledge.

Dimitrijević, A., Frankel, J. B., & Cassullo, G. (Eds.) (2018). *Sándor Ferenczi's Influence on Contemporary Psychoanalytic Traditions*. London: Karnac.

Falzeder, E. (2015). *Psychoanalytic Filiations: Mapping the Psychoanalytic Movement*. Abingdon, UK: Routledge, 2019.

Ferenczi, S. (1913). CG Jung, Wandlungen und Symbole der Libido. Beiträge zur Entwicklungsgeschichte des Denkens. *Internationale Zeitschrift für Psychoanalyse*, *1*(4): 391–403.

Ferenczi, S. (1949). Confusion of the tongues between the adults and the child—(The language of tenderness and of passion). *International Journal of Psychoanalysis*, *30*(4): 225–230.

Ferenczi, S. (1988). *The Clinical Diary of Sándor Ferenczi*, J. Dupont (Ed.). Cambridge, MA: Harvard University Press.

Ferenczi, S., & Rank, O. (1924). *The Development of Psychoanalysis.* New York: Nervous and Mental Disease Publishing Co., 1925.

Freud, S. (1900a). *The Interpretation of Dreams. S. E.*, *4–5*: ix–627. London: Hogarth.

Freud, S. (1901b). *The Psychopathology of Everyday Life. S. E.*, *6*: vii–296. London: Hogarth.

Freud, S. (1910a). Five lectures on psycho-analysis. *S. E.*, *11*: 1–56. London: Hogarth.

Freud, S. (1910k). "Wild" psycho-analysis. *S. E.*, *11*: 219–228. London: Hogarth.

Freud, S. (1914d). On the history of the psycho-analytic movement. *S. E.*, *14*: 1–66. London: Hogarth.

Freud, S. (1925d). *An Autobiographical Study. S. E.*, *20*: 1–74. London: Hogarth.

Freud, S. (1926d). *Inhibitions, Symptoms and Anxiety. S. E.*, *20*: 75–176. London: Hogarth.

Grosskurth, P. (1991). *The Secret Ring: Freud's Inner Circle and the Politics of Psychoanalysis.* Reading, MA: Addison-Wesley/Longman.

Habarth, J., Hansell, J., & Grove, T. (2011). How accurately do introductory psychology textbooks present psychoanalytic theory? *Teaching of Psychology*, *38*(1): 16–21.

Holmes, J. (1993). *John Bowlby and Attachment Theory.* London: Routledge, 2014.

Hornstein, G. A. (1992). The return of the repressed: Psychology's problematic relations with psychoanalysis, 1909–1960. *American Psychologist*, *47*(2): 254–263.

Hornstein, G. A. (2000). *To Redeem One Person Is to Redeem the World: A Life of Frieda Fromm-Reichmann.* New York: Simon & Schuster.

Janus, L. (2010). Die "Technik der Psychoanalyse" von Otto Rank. Eine Ressource für die heutige Psychoanalyse. *Forum der Psychoanalyse*, *26*: 129–150.

Janus, L. (2014). Otto Rank: Der Mensch als Künstler—Kreativität als Wesenskern des Menschen. In: G. Gödde & J. Zirfas (Eds.), *Lebenskunst im 20. Jahrhundert. Stimmen von Philosophen, Künstlern und Therapeuten* (pp. 303–320). Munich, Germany: Wilhelm Fink Verlag.

Kernberg, O. F. (1986). Institutional problems of psychoanalytic education. *Journal of the American Psychoanalytic Association*, 34: 799–834.

Kernberg, O. F. (1992). Authoritarianism, culture, and personality in psychoanalytic education. *Journal of the International Association for the History of Psychoanalysis*, 5: 341–354.

Kernberg, O. F. (1996). Thirty methods to destroy the creativity of psychoanalytic candidates. *International Journal of Psychoanalysis*, 77(5): 1031–1040.

Kernberg, O. F. (2000). A concerned critique of psychoanalytic education. *International Journal of Psychoanalysis*, 81: 97–120.

Kernberg, O. F. (2012). Suicide prevention for psychoanalytic institutes and societies. *Journal of the American Psychoanalytic Association*, 60(4): 707–719.

Kirsch, M., Dimitrijević, A., & Buchholz, M. B. (2022). "Death drive" scientifically reconsidered. *Frontiers in Psychology*. DOI: 10.3389/fpsyg. 2022.941328.

Kohut, H. (1959). Introspection, empathy, and psychoanalysis an examination of the relationship between mode of observation and theory. *Journal of the American Psychoanalytic Association*, 7(3): 459–483.

Kohut, H. (1981). On empathy. *International Journal of Psychoanalytic Self Psychology*, 5(2): 122–131.

Kohut, H. (1982). Introspection, empathy, and the semi-circle of mental health. *International Journal of Psychoanalysis*, 63: 395–407.

Kuhn, P. (2002a). "Romancing with a wealth of detail". Narratives of Ernest Jones's 1906 trial for indecent assault. *Studies in Gender and Sexuality*, 3(4): 344–378.

Kuhn, P. (2002b). So, if it were not Jones, who else would it be? Reply to commentaries. *Studies in Gender and Sexuality*, 3(4): 395–405.

Kuhn, P. (2014a). Footnotes in the history of British psychoanalysis: Observing Ernest Jones discerning the works of Sigmund Freud, 1905–1908. *Psychoanalysis and History*, 16(1): 5–54.

Kuhn, P. (2014b). Subterranean histories: The dissemination of Freud's works into the British discourse on psychological medicine, 1904–1911. *Psychoanalysis and History*, 16(2): 153–214.

Kuhn, P. (2015). In 'The Dark Regions of the Mind'. A reading for the indecent assault in Ernest Jones's 1908 dismissal from the West End Hospital for Nervous Diseases. *Psychoanalysis and History, 17*(1): 7–57.

Makari, G. (2008). *Revolution in Mind: The Creation of Psychoanalysis.* New York: Harper Collins.

Masson, J. M. (1985). *The Assault on Truth: Freud's Suppression of the Seduction Theory.* London: Faber.

Mitchell, S. A. (1991). Editorial philosophy. *Psychoanalytic Dialogues, 1*: 1–7.

Nitzschke, B. (1992). … im Interesse unserer psychoanalytischen Sache in Deutschland. In: J. Wiesse (Ed.), *Chaos und Regel.* Göttingen, Germany: Vandenhoeck & Ruprecht.

Park, S. W. (2006). Psychoanalysis in textbooks of introductory psychology: A review. *Journal of the American Psychoanalytic Association, 54*(4): 1361–1380.

Peglau, A. (2013). Unpolitische Wissenschaft? Wilhelm Reich und die Psychoanalyse im Nationalsozialismus. *Bibliothek der Psychoanalyse.* Gießen, Germany: Psychosozial-Verlag.

Rank, O. (1924). The trauma of birth in its importance for psychoanalytic therapy. *Psychoanalytic Review, 11*: 241–245.

Rubin, L. R. (2002). Wilhelm Reich and Anna Freud: His expulsion from psychoanalysis. *International Forum of Psychoanalysis, 12*: 109–117.

Rudnytsky, P. L. (2002). *Reading Psychoanalysis: Freud, Rank, Ferenczi, Groddeck.* Ithaka, NY: Cornell University Press.

Rudnytsky, P. L. (2011). *Rescuing Psychoanalysis from Freud and Other Essays in Re-Vision.* New York: Routledge.

Rudnytsky, P. L. (2019). *Formulated Experiences: Hidden Realities and Emergent Meanings From Shakespeare to Fromm.* New York: Routledge.

Siegel, P., Josephs, L., & Weinberger, J. (2002). Where's the text? The problem of validation in psychoanalysis. *Journal of the American Psychoanalytic Association, 50*: 407–428.

Silver, A. L. (2018). Psychoanalysis and psychosis: Ferenczi's influence at Chestnut Lodge. In: A. Dimitriejvic, G. Cassullo, & J. B. Frankel (Eds.), *Ferenczi's Influence on Contemporary Psychoanalytic Traditions* (pp. 213–219). London: Routledge.

Stefana, A., Celentani, B., Dimitrijević, A., Migone, P., & Albasi, C. (2021). Where is psychoanalysis today? Sixty-two psychoanalysts share their subjective perspectives on the state of the art of psychoanalysis: A qualitative thematic analysis. *International Forum of Psychoanalysis, 30*(4): 234–246. https://doi.org/10.1080/0803706X.2021.1991594.

Stepansky, P. E. (2009). *Psychoanalysis at the Margins.* New York: Other Press.

Wallerstein, R. S. (2004). From dissidence to pluralism in psychoanalysis—and onto what? In: M. S. Bergmann (Ed.), *Understanding Dissidence and Controversy in the History of Psychoanalysis* (pp. 201–228). New York: Other Press.

Winthuis, B. (2006). Otto Rank und "Der Mythus von der Geburt des Helden". *Jahrbuch für Gruppenanalyse, 12*: 169–185.

Wittenberger, G. (1988). Die Geschichte des "Geheimen Komitees". Psychoanalyse im Institutionalisierungsprozeß. *Psyche—Zeitschrift Für Psychoanalyse und Ihre Anwendungen, 42*: 44–52.

Zweig, M. B. (1971). Wilhelm Reich's theory: Ethical implications. *American Imago, 28*(3): 268–286.

CHAPTER 10

Examples of silencing in the psychotherapy office

Aleksandar Dimitrijević

I cannot count the number of patients who have mentioned the feeling of inability, or the lack of daring, to share important emotions, experiences, and attitudes with anyone around them. "Different! Always different!"—I have heard those cries so many times that I believe every psychotherapist must be dealing with them regularly. One person claimed to be the only non-right-wing member of his work unit and could not decide what was more frustrating: to remain silent and betray his conviction or to speak up and risk bullying or even being beaten up. Another felt no one could understand his artistic and philosophical interests, and people ridiculed him because he was intellectually superior. Women who accepted themselves as attractive had lost faith that anyone would ever truly listen to what they might have to say; women who considered themselves unattractive despaired that it was useless to talk, and everyone listened only because they were not pretty. Many were afraid that being honest might lead to political persecution. Almost everyone married or in a relationship had a secret they felt would destroy the relationship if revealed. Some ran away from the pressure of religions that put other people's words in their mouths and gave up "looking for your own way". Several needed years of therapy to emancipate themselves from parents who claimed to know everything better and wanted to guide them through life even when the patients were in their thirties and forties. Once I started paying attention to this, I became convinced that the essential thing we do as psychotherapists is helping people voice silenced parts of their personalities.

Silencing in the psychiatric hospital

My first job as a psychologist was at a psychiatric hospital, in a female ward, where around ninety women spent between several weeks and several months. Officially, it was a "chronic psychosis" unit, with all the prison elements that such institutions include. In reality, at least one out of every three patients was there because of poverty, hunger, cold, etc.

The primary thing that was expected of me was to write reports about psychological assessment procedures—Wechsler scales, Rorschach ink-blots, and the like. However, I soon started noticing that interviews were full of trauma, violence, and rape, while most medical records did not say a word about that. So, I started enquiring, and patient after patient replied, "No one ever asked me about this," even though some had been repeatedly hospitalised for years, sometimes decades, one even since before I was born.

What were the victims doing about all these experiences? In a nutshell, nothing. They had no hope that anything could change and just made this "don't ask, don't tell" a routine of their lives. Many simply said, "He is my husband." One explained, "I go to the stables and beat horses and cows" (the reason for this probably being that cattle have no words for pain either). Frequent were also the explanations that protest was impossible because of poverty, unemployment, and the lack of support.

I felt the most painful part of all this was that as professionals, we were not only unfocused on this problem, but the system was not even aware of its existence.

"Don't ever tell this to your father!"

When I met Alfred, he was almost forty. Successful, married, with three children, he lived in one of the most comfortable neighbourhoods of Berlin. He had never been in psychotherapy before and came to see me only after his GP repeatedly advised him. He waited for his turn for more than three months, but even then had no idea how I could help him.

The only problem I have is medical. I have abdominal problems. I have already had one haemorrhoid operation, and I have frequent digestion problems. So, it is mostly constipation, gases, and such stuff. But even a colonoscopy couldn't find anything, so I don't know how psychotherapy can be of help.

Several minutes later, we turned to his childhood reminiscences. He seemed glad to talk about that. When he was about seven, it turned out, his father went to work abroad, and his mother befriended a neighbouring family. There was a fifteen-year-old boy there who invited Alfred and his younger sister to play in his bed with the lights off. For two years, no one noticed anything.

One day, Alfred felt strong enough to resist going there and managed to take his sister and himself out of the abuse. I thought it was too early for me to ask him whether that included penetration, for which colonoscopy would be a repetition.

Only months after this salvation, he felt strong enough to start talking to his mother.

> I still remember that vividly. I was in the kitchen, and she worked on something. I was crying. I had to lean against the wall. The strength had disappeared. But I told her everything. She turned, and looked at me intently, but remained silent. Then, suddenly, she said, "Don't ever tell this to your father! He will divorce me!" Then I went silent, and she returned to cooking. After that, we never spoke about this again.

His wife of ten years also didn't know anything about this, and he had only recently opened the topic with his sister. And although he spoke to me so openly, he never came to his scheduled sessions again.

Wordless crying

It was not until I started writing notes that I realised how stupid I had been. Why did I think "domestic abuse" referred to Ute's mother and not her? There would be no reason for her to be in psychotherapy for most of her childhood if she was not the molested one. So why did I not enquire?

In the coming sessions, I figured out there was nothing stupid about that. Ute grew up to be a master in coming across as sociable, cheerful, competent, and resilient. I did not see her as a once traumatised child, just as her colleagues, friends, and lovers did not.

But where did this all come from? Before she even started school, her father had not only touched her inappropriately but used a mind-twisting threat: "Do not mention this to anyone! I have put little people in your room, and they will let me know if you tell anyone!" There were nights when she would go to her mother's room, crying her eyes out but not dare say a word. Her anguish was understood only by her desperate refusals to spend the weekends at her father's place. But she kept doing her best to never tell anyone around her. Then, as well as now.

Silent to avoid ridicule

Bruce came to me deeply worried about himself. Like everyone else nowadays, he googled medical terms and gave himself a diagnosis. His interpretation was that he was "borderline". His specific complaints were fear of people, awkwardness, and insecurity in social situations, sometimes coupled with bouts of anger, quarrels, and endless heated debates. He lived alone and left the apartment only when he had to. Worst of all, he complained about facing constant pressure from his parents. Looking at him, so youthful at the age of twenty-seven, very tall and skinny, I didn't find that difficult to imagine. Still, I asked.

> My parents think that I cannot take care of myself, especially when it comes to social situations. They call me every day, ask about everything and then criticise me. If you ask them, I never do anything right. They think I don't understand people and that I hallucinate things. So, I always hesitate to talk to people, afraid they will laugh at me when I say something crazy.

Immediately, I wanted to know more. This sounded too bizarre compared to the person I was looking at.

He explained that since his childhood, his parents accused him of "inventing stories". If he spoke about their punishments, for example, they would laugh and say, "What makes you imagine such things!?" He claimed this happened regularly, possibly once a week when he was a child and more often now. And I thought his parents had destroyed his trust in his mind, and he never learned how to make friends because he worked hard on silencing the mind he thought was "crazy". But I could not say that so early in the treatment.

Silenced emotions

A brief enquiry provided only the most basic information: thirty-two, Korean, dancer. But the name meant nothing to me, and I still had no idea how to be of help.

When I opened the conversation, he asked me, "What are emotions? And where can I find them?" I asked him to explain what he meant and why that was important. Not that I wanted to deflect his questions, I was just intrigued by the pseudo scientific tone in the therapy room.

J. had moved to Berlin several months earlier to work with a renowned choreographer but discovered his ineptitude. The work was stuck because he (J.), in the words of the other guy, French in origin, was "empty": "You move your arms and legs, but there are no emotions in you!" So, not to lose this tremendous opportunity, he thought the best person to help him find these "emotions" must be a psychologist.

Yes, he had to agree, he probably had no emotions. Or he just had no idea what they were or how to recognise them. He was never sad, angry, or jealous. ("Are these the emotions?") Truth be told, he used to feel them long ago:

> As a small boy, I cried several times and protested. But each time, my parents' faces would remain completely the same, and my father, dead serious, would only say: "Why is it that you don't respect me?"

"What did he mean by that," I asked naively, utterly unaware of the context. The society in his home country, I was told, was strictly hierarchical, and children were at the bottom of the family ladder of power. Therefore, they were expected to execute the orders without any reactions or comments, least of all emotions. And some of them remained silenced for life.

It remains a mystery to me whether his descriptions of his culture and language were correct.

Silenced burns

Bianca wrote to me because her mother suggested she should do so. Herself, she had no idea whether that made sense. Whenever she was supposed to make a decision, she consulted her mother. After each date, she called her mother, described all the details, and learned whether that was "the right boyfriend for her". With disarming honesty, she told me that she had no opinions, tastes, interests, or hobbies. Luckily, she believed, she had "such a wise, perfect mother" to get advice from.

Yes, she has always felt like this. One of the earliest things she could remember shows how much she loved her mother. When she was around six years of age, during their summer vacation, her mother prepared tea and accidentally spilt the whole pot of boiling water over Bianca's legs.

> It hurt horribly. I have never felt such pain again in my life. They took me to the hospital, and doctors forbade me from swimming. But I knew I must not cry or complain. I had to protect my mother and not allow guilt to take her away from me.

Mother's love was precious, and the clever girl noticed she could quickly lose it if the mother got overwhelmed by guilt or was not offered the sacrifice of endless praise. So, the heavy price Bianca paid was that she completely stifled her childhood voices, and then she never looked for the adult ones.

"Adults always know better"

Preparing invoices is possibly the most tedious part of the psychotherapist's job. I have always tried to do that as fast as possible, copy, paste, change the date and, if necessary, the amount. Done this hundreds of times, if not more.

One day I received a cautious, almost anxious question about one of my invoices. Complete with details of which dates, how many sessions, and the total amount. I saw it very late in the evening and did not understand where the problem was. I opened the attached document and discovered that I indeed had made a mistake—I sent the invoice from two months ago without any changes. Only the names were correct.

But what was I to do now? To apologise immediately was easy, so was sending the corrected invoice early the next day. The next session was what puzzled me.

I decided to take the lead at the opening and suggested that we talk about what happened. Giulia told me she had received my initial message around 11 a.m. and spent the early afternoon drafting and redrafting her possible reply. Her memory seemed clear, but it was difficult to trust it when my invoice claimed we had had one session more than she believed. When she thought about that on her own, she held she was right. However, when she considered telling me this, she froze in horror. She was sure I would get offended, point to her mistake, and refuse to continue her therapy. "Adults", said this thirty-year-old woman, "always know better, and I should better shut up because I can only anger them."

Self-imposed silence

One patient described one conversation from twenty-five years ago with these words:

> Mother took me out of the house. We crossed the road. I had no idea why. We stood on the lawn. "Could play soccer here?" I thought. She told me she would have to travel for work and therefore, wouldn't be home for a year. "I will miss her," I thought. She said I could call her. Dad would take care of me. She would be back soon. I didn't say anything. I knew she was leaving because of their constant fights. I knew she would never come back. But I felt too sorry for her to tell her she was lying. Who can feel better after being called a liar by an eight year old?

Silencing desires

Adam was quite successful in many domains and rather popular. He felt miserable, though, when it came to the expectation to start a family. It was not easy for him to fall in love, and he found his sex life "moderate, not bad, but not exciting either". Now, in the last couple of months, there was a new girl whom he found very attractive, but she wanted adventure.

He didn't want to lose her, and still, he didn't care about any of her sugges-tions. She called him "Vanilla Ice", contemptuously, he believed. He tried to be rough, but that gave him nothing but a panic attack.

In psychotherapy, he would only go one step at a time. Then the girl left, and his confidence and optimism evaporated. Slowly, I learned that he came from a strict Catholic background. He was the only child and grew up with his mother, father having died when Adam was too young to even remember him.

Much later, he mentioned having a girlfriend when he was sixteen. It began as a naive, childhood crush. Then one evening, his mother said solemnly, "Other men can do that. But not you. You're better than that." He broke it up the next day.

Not for anything in the world would he risk losing his mother's love and respect. Not even for the call of his youthful desires and needs. Years passed, and he moved to another continent. Women liked him pretty much. Still, his mother's voice resounded in his mind, while his "sinful" side was still silenced and tame.

These were, of course, just my thoughts. We were ages away from connecting these things in our dialogues.

"Lips glued, tongue swollen"

Our native languages have no similarities whatsoever, and without Eng-lish, we would not be able to understand a word of what the other one is saying. Yet, Frieda was coming to sessions regularly, before I even under-stood the problem in its entirety. She did her best to avoid any conflict and was shy in expressing her opinions beyond a small circle of her friends. Finally, one day she gathered strength and told me it was the same with me during sessions. She was horrified by the idea of "saying whatever comes to your mind first", which I had invited her to do. She admitted that all the time, she was coming to sessions with an already well-thought-out material, almost an agenda. She also liked talking about dreams because, here as well, she was coming up with an elaborate story. When I did not say anything to her, she remained silent for about five minutes. "That was a frightening experience," she finally said. At every impulse to say some-thing spontaneously, she felt "her lips were glued, and her tongue swol-len". She then returned to silence until the time for that session was up.

Silencing through talking too much

There are, also, patients who talk too much without purpose. Not rude, not disrespectful, just incapable of receiving much (or anything for that matter) from the therapist. So, they silence the supposed source of help and pay to receive almost nothing. Indeed, resistance can be summoned to make the proverbial silent analyst completely silent.

One person spoke so much about her work, three times a week, I was hardly able to carve out a moment to say a couple of words. Wrestling with boredom, I had to point out this several times before we could think about it.

In my experience, men, incomparably more often than women, tell jokes or would rather just chat than dive into the painful domain of emotional life. Some women, on the other hand, rather spend the whole session portraying other people (sometimes with captivating storytelling abilities and psychological insight) and refuse to admit that this makes it impossible to focus on their actual pain during therapy.

Somewhat more obviously, patients may directly reject what we are trying to tell them. I remember more than one patient who would interrupt me in the middle of a sentence whenever I wanted to ask for clarification related to his/her parents, spouses, or children, and continue talking about something less personal for a long time.

Silencing unacceptable emotions

Manuela came to me after her boss suggested she should look for psychotherapy. There was a clear trigger for that. She became emotional at work, and when that was pointed out she grew even more emotional. She even cried before several of her colleagues.

She does not get emotional often. Quite opposite to that experience, she is professional, effective, and excels at multitasking. And does not even mention having a private life, I could have added.

So, it all started when in the middle of a meeting she was accused of being too protective of her team. A colleague, not a superior, did not allow her to speak, yelled at her, and seeing her reaction said, "And now you are getting emotional! Typical!"

— How did he say that? What did his tone sound like?
— Angry. Contemptuous. Dismissive. Belittling.
— Aren't these emotions too?
— Well, yes. But these are acceptable emotions.
— What makes them acceptable?
— These are male emotions and men have decided they are acceptable. Whereas my emotions are feminine and soft, and they do not belong in the conference room.

Immediately the next day, I received an email from her. She wrote, "I thank you for the session, it was enormously helpful. I spoke with several female colleagues, and they all confirmed my experience. I feel much better. I have understood I do not need psychotherapy; I am not crazy. So, I would like to cancel the next session and the whole therapy."

She never contacted me again. Therefore, I am still curious whether she changed her work environment, or fought against attempts to silence her.

I also had to silence my opinion that she probably needed therapy very much but for an opposite reason to what had triggered her boss to suggest therapy.

Silencing imperfections

With each new client, I want to know how he or she got their name. Who chose it, is there a family story related to it, and what is the meaning of it in their native language? Many times, I would eventually understand that the whole problem started with the choice of the name.

There is hardly any other name as burdensome as Angela. It sounds nice in different languages and different forms. It brings the association that good news is about to arrive. But the girl can feel that what is expected of her is perfection, maybe even supernatural perfection. Maybe the parents chose that name because they were not able to bear their sense of imperfection.

Angela who felt this most acutely was even older than I, but still constantly concerned about other people's opinions about her. "But then I'm afraid they won't like me," she repeated time and again. She was helpful, a perfect hostess, understanding, friendly, and humorous—an angel.

At the same time, she believed that people, outside therapy sessions, did not like anger, sadness, pessimism, complaints, and so on. "I know that these are perfectly normal emotions when I see them in other people. But when I feel them, I call them negative emotions, and I try to hide them from other people."

Sometimes, when she would try to share some of these experiences, she would end up disappointed. She was afraid of creating boundaries at work, and she did not know how to cry in the presence of another person, which would make her return to her silenced loneliness and the habituated pleasing behaviour.

CHAPTER 11

Dream-telling in family therapy sessions: how they can change silencing into hearables

Michael B. Buchholz

Introduction

Many psychoanalytic authors have observed the after-effects of traumas in dreams and dream analysis, while others have described the after-effects of traumas in the next generations. It is rare to find the combination of dream-telling and dream analysis in family therapy sessions to better understand the role and mechanisms of intergenerational exchange and traditions held (Buchholz, 1990b; Danieli, 2006; Graaf, 1998). In my therapeutic life, as head of an educational counselling centre and later as a member of an academic family research centre, I worked with many families. One of my academic aims was to show how to apply the psychoanalytic method in the family therapy (Buchholz, 1982) and I later described a triangular approach to the family therapy (Buchholz, 1990a). Furthermore, I was running debates with colleagues from a systemic orientation, which has taught me a lot. Here I present clinical examples of family sessions.

A history of family accidents

When ten-year-old Torsten started talking about hanging himself, his family was alarmed and sought out therapy. In the ninth session, the mother addressed the fear which was prominent in the family. Torsten regularly used to wake up at night from anxiety dreams with piercing screams. Since the birth of his now eight-year-old sister Nora, Torsten was constantly sick, and his mother spent a lot of time at the doctor's. She felt annoyed by him and his stubbornness; the daily school home-work was torture, and his school performance was abysmal. The father, a farmer, would retreat to the fields because he wanted nothing to do with the domestic "nagging".

The previous sessions had somewhat calmed the sibling conflict. The powerful erotic attraction between Torsten and Nora had become apparent as they both often played husband and wife in the evenings. However, if there was a quarrel, no one was on Torsten's side; he was always in the wrong. So, it was no wonder that Torsten "didn't want to live anymore" and threatened to hang himself.

A dream session

In the ninth session, the father was able to recall that he had been "con-stantly beaten" as a child and had not been able to find "any real courage to live at all". He also sometimes cried loudly at night. This enabled Torsten to talk about his strange dreams. He dreamt that the cows had run away, and he had to catch them again. Even though he could not catch them, he had to keep running after them, resulting in him wak-ing up in fear. After recounting this dream, he remembers another one where he builds a snowman and then breaks it again. Now, Nora also remembers something she dreamt: an assassin with a poison syringe is chasing her, and she has to run away. She wakes up terrified. The mother reacts saying she can't remember any of her dreams lately, but she used to have similar ones to Nora: a murderer "with a gun or something" was running after her and she had to run away. "Sweat was running down my whole body," she says.

The family is shaken by this sudden outbreak of a dream series, which seems to respond to one another. Nora follows Torsten; their rela-tionship has "poisoned" aspects. Torsten overpowers her sometimes.

Their fear of being slaughtered like cows corresponds to the regressive symbol formation of integrity threatened by early sexual attacks. Violence and love combine in a traumatising way, which comes up in other interpretative stories of their dreams.

Torsten, the mother says, is afraid when she and her husband go out in the evening. Nora adds, "I can imagine that when you go out in the evening, Torsten thinks you're going to have an accident." The parents did have a traffic accident a few months ago. When Torsten found out about it, Nora recalls that he "really collapsed" and Torsten screams: "That's not true!" The mother explains that when Torsten rides away on his bike, Nora yells that she's afraid something will happen to him. The fearful mother then drives after him.

I say to the family that all these dreams seem to have something in common. They were all about leaving: the father goes to the field, the cows run away, and the mother has to run away from a murderer. All of them are afraid, but all of them also did something threatening: Torsten screams at night, which frightens the mother; Torsten feels threatened by tasks he can't handle—at school and herding the cows in the dream; he also breaks something, the snowman in the dream. In real life something threatening did happen, the parents had an accident, and the children feel threateningly left alone when the parents leave—there would be both: a lot of fear, but sometimes also something that scares them.

The family is silent.

Then the mother reopens the conversation and tells them about her fears for Torsten. She helps him with his homework, but she always gets upset: "I would like to pull Torsten to me and push him away at the same time." After a pause, she adds, quite startled, "When he's good, I want to pull him to me. When he's bad, I want to push him away."

When I say that it's as if there are two Torstens, one good and one bad, she says emotionally, "That's true. Sometimes … I would like to … strangle him," she hesitates for a long time.

The tenth session

The mother opens with a message she has been thinking about for a long time: already as a child, she had to take care of her bedridden mother for many years. She managed the household and carried out all the disgusting tasks connected with the care without grumbling—but during this time she dreamt of the nightly murderers. In daydreams, she imagined that one day she would lead a more pleasant life on a farm, but her son, Torsten, seemed to her like a continuation of all these burdens. She transferred all her hopes onto him and was bitter when Torsten did not live up to them. Then he was "bad", and she pushed him away.

As we talk about it, with the three other family members listening very attentively, I learn that she also had a very conflictual relationship with her brother who was two years older than her. He was preferred by her parents and even inherited the parental farm, while she had sacrificed herself so much caring for her mother! Furthermore, another brother, seven years older, had died of diphtheria when she was two years old. He was supposed to inherit the farm. Her surviving brother became a farmer and owner of the parental farm. She broke all ties with him.

The opening of this highly conflictual transgenerational perspective in the mother's self-reflection shakes the other family members and me as well.

The eleventh session

The family brings along the seventy-six-year-old "grandpa", the father of Torsten's father. This was not arranged; grandfather had been told about the sessions and now he wanted to be there for once.

He lived in the house, and it was said that there was often a "quarrel" with him because he stood by Torsten. In response to my query, he immediately shared his reason willingly: his oldest son, the six years older brother of Torsten's father, drowned at the age of six while playing at a fire pond in which water is stored for firefighting. Mr J., therefore, owes his takeover of the family farm to the fact that his brother had an accident and died.

The idea that the eldest son must die runs through generations, hence the conscious anxious concern for Torsten today. The dream of the cows running away reveals further meaning: why does Torsten have to catch fleeing cows; would that not be the father's task? The answer comes if we understand the dream as Torsten's conception of grandiosity and omnipotence. In the dream, the father is "not there", and Torsten can dreamingly imagine taking over the farm. He is alarmed and wakes up when he realises that he cannot manage this task. The father supports him in imagining that one does not need to know any academic things to take over the farm. The decisive factor is whether he can drive a tractor.

Towards the end of this session, I told Torsten that he must have had a hard time. Following his father and not taking school things seriously brings him into conflict with his mother, who spends a lot of time with him on his homework and wants him to take it seriously. She (the mother) experiences a similar frustration with this as she did when she was caring for her mother. But Torsten is also a part of another family tradition: oldest sons, it seems, are expected to "disappear", and the family came to me because they were so frightened when Torsten talked about hanging himself. Torsten cried with relief, Nora gave me a friendly look—and the grandfather beamed, saying, "This is how they should have talked in [his] family years ago!". Two weeks later in the next session, Torsten brought his maths notebook from school. He had a top grade—I was relieved, and also a bit happy, considering the stress of this treatment.

Reflections

I have described here a "relationship trap" whose transgenerational aspects have become clearer. I have always been surprised that the early concept of the "double bind" (Bateson, 1978) has disappeared from family therapy discourse; my experience is that it is very useful for understanding family dramas, including that dreams and a transgenerational perspective show, however, such double binds are of a higher complexity, but they are still double binds. For a child to follow his father's expectations (driving a tractor) *or* his mother's (doing homework) is an unsolvable task. As it is to follow the father's and grandfather's tradition of the fate of the eldest son, or the mother's tradition who sacrificed her life for her mother? Questions of that kind are not asked, and missing answers constitute the silencing of children who impress us with serious threats like committing suicide. It is not repetition compulsion, a concept which would make the therapeutic task unsolvable. It is the therapeutic reflection of unthought but real traditions and their power, which can be heard in family sessions—and made hearable. Telling dreams not only to the analyst but in the presence of those who play a role in them, helps to hear the silenced distress of a child, like Torsten. The powerful voices of those who silence must in turn consent so that what is silenced can leave the mode of helpless symptomatic cries and enter the field of meaningful communication.

A murderous family

After a suicide attempt (with sleeping pills) and a subsequent stay in a psychiatric ward, Vicky, sixteen, has been referred to family therapy. She is the only daughter of a wealthy businessman and his wife. The suicide attempt was preceded by severe, physical altercations with the father. The father would not tolerate Vicky's relationships with young men and as a result locked her in her room, beat her severely, and controlled her every move, sometimes with the help of others. The mother is very depressed and regularly takes sedative medication (which Vicky helped herself to). She did not try, as is often the case, to protect Vicky from her father's assaults.

For a long time, Vicky's relationship with a southern European worker remained secret. But when it came out that the father had had a girlfriend for years, she triumphantly told him about her own new experiences. This led to serious arguments, which led to her taking the pills. The parents do not understand why Vicky had to do this; they mainly blame her for making the family the talk of the small town.

Vicky's dream report

In the fourth session Vicky reports a dream: "In a forest or bushes, I find a bird's nest that somehow fell on the ground. When I go to pick it up, there's an egg inside, and it's broken in half. I keep telling myself, 'Throw it away, the old thing,' but somehow, I can't, I have it in my hand and I can't throw it away. I don't understand that."

The family becomes very quiet for a minute and a half after Vicky tells this dream. Then something unexpected happens: the father, this hard, big man, starts to cry! When he is finally able to speak, he says to his daughter in amazing clairvoyance: "This throwing away of something that belongs to you, after all, is so hard, so cold, so ... so ... so merciless." He understands the dream as if Vicky wanted to throw herself away; then the broken egg would be an experiential symbol for herself.

Vicky bursts out in rage: "This throwaway mentality was your own." At that time, he had dismissed several employees of the company, not caring how they would continue to fare. She had been sent to a spa when she was four years old. Although, as it turned out, it was only one of several medical options. Hardness? He certainly did not need to reproach her for that! He had beaten her often enough. For the first time, the mother cautiously joined her daughter: it was he who had decided to give little Vicky away for a cure; she had already said at the time that she was not in favour of it. With the beatings as well, she adds quietly, she had never agreed!

Details of a transgenerational trauma

The father first wants to intervene against the mother's new coalition, but then comes to his senses and tries to explain that he had been severely beaten by his mother. Only when his older brother died in a traffic accident did it become clear that he would take over the company. Even though his relationship with his parents had improved somewhat, he was always full of revenge. After a serious altercation with his father in the cellar, he was on the verge of beating him to death with a hatchet. He left the house in a hurry and never wanted to see his parents again. He became a sailor for many years and only returned home when he heard that his father had died. He took over the business and covered all traces that could have pointed to his father. He had already become very hard.

And then the mother asks him, "And what about that accident?" I sense the disclosure of a terrible secret is brewing. "Do we really want to talk about it?" the father asks, his eyes sharply fixed on his wife. "Yes," the mother answers simply, but also so tersely that she suddenly allows no argument. When Vicky was three years old, the family owned a motorboat. Once, while driving, the mother jumped into the water and the father at the wheel made a turn at that moment, so that by a hair's breadth the mother would have been caught by the spinning propeller. She sustained a minor injury to her leg. She always took it as an attempted murder, and when she found out that he had already had a girlfriend at that time, it was another confirmation that he had wanted to get rid of her.

The family created an atmosphere that made me hold my breath.

Yes, says the father, he often thought it would be good if she were not there and he hated her with a passion. But at that time? No, he did not want to kill her. He admitted his hatred for his wife. She had interfered with his business plans at the time. She had plotted against him with his employees—the ones he then fired. The mother also confirmed this, saying she also hated him and had schemed against him.

Traumatic over-effects

Vicky did not know that this incident preceded her being sent to the spa. Upon realising this she starts to cry.

At this point, I say to her, "The dream represents the domestic nest that was destroyed very early. The egg, like you, is broken in half, as if one half should belong to the father, the other half to the mother." Vicky replies, "And then a chick can't survive well." "That's right," I continue the dialogue with Vicky (noting how both parents are listening), "you seem to be trying to break away from this parent, somewhat violently yourself, trying to shake this nest from your hand; and at the same time, you seem to feel that the chick needs to be protected for now, and in doing so, you've taken on the rather difficult task of trying to bring the parents together so that the two halves of the egg can also heal back together." Vicky answers: "I am once large, but then somehow empty, and I must be large so that sometime in the future perhaps, I can be small again. But actually, that's not possible at all!"

I conclude this case report with the information that after two further sessions I recommended Vicky turn to individual therapy for herself, which she accepted. A few years later, I received a letter from her wherein she thanked me for these family sessions, "They opened my eyes and soul," she wrote. My proposal for the parents to think about marriage therapy was not accepted, and they divorced.

Some reflections

I had recently read Mary-Joan Gerson's book *The Embedded Self* which was about psychoanalytic family therapy (Gerson, 1996). Vicky presented her dream *as if* she had read the book, too. Her dream shows the lack of embeddedness she suffered from.

What does the fact say, that she could have this dream and report it in the session with her parents present? To answer this question, it is useful to be aware of the difference between concreteness and metaphor. The discussion of the dream leads initially—through the father's remark that the egg is Vicky herself—to a metaphorical level. It is quickly abandoned and leads to the discussion about the family's relationship with violence. These are not dreams, but concrete in a brutal way. In this way, the "egg-break" becomes understandable, one level explaining the other. But the metaphor of the broken egg which the dream creates is a genuinely creative psychic achievement of Vicky's: the dream is a cry for help addressed to the therapist to perceive the broken self.

There is a discontinuity between the dream and the family drama: the dream does not dissolve in the family history; it is a creation in itself which sheds light onto family life and its consequences hoping that the metaphor will be understood in its hard reality. Through this discontinuity, the psyche, as it were, illustrates itself. Vicky's dream representation seeks to bring herself to the view of the parents and the therapist, and here, the father can empathise with the first remark based on his biography. He thus succeeds in the first interpretation of the dream, although it might not be more than a projection. Vicky presents herself to the father with the dream and it succeeds: the father recognises her, and thereby, from another perspective, recognises himself. It is this process of mutual recognition that the family therapist has to support.

A dream without the dreamer

A couple came to their second meeting without their ten-year-old son Klaus. He was on a country school trip. Immediately after the explanation of his absence, Mrs L. said that Klaus had dreamt of a spider, a large and horrible animal. He had slept very restlessly and fearfully. When she tried to comfort him, he pushed her away. Mrs L. began to cry: "A spider claws like this, and I also claw like this sometimes, and a spider is so voracious ..." She pauses and explains that she sees herself in this spider and is shocked that Klaus is afraid of her.

Klaus was missing in this session, but the dream was a message that represented him. I learned that the ten-year-old boy had been sleeping next to his mother when his father hadn't been home a few weeks ago because of a business trip. Therefore, Klaus had this dream in bed next to his mother.

Psychoanalysts interpret the spider as a dream symbol for the mother (Abraham, 1923), even though completely different interpretations have been proposed (Rohde-Dachser, 2016). Where does the mother get the certainty that she is the spider? My answer is that she doesn't know but behaves in her *action of telling* the dream as if she is "clawing". She makes Klaus's dream her own.

The content of a narrative is something different from the *action of telling*. The *narrative* self or *told self* is dramatically presentable and audible; the *telling* self, on the other hand, cannot reflect during the telling and is, in this sense, unconscious (Deppermann et al., 2020).

The telling of the dream is thus associated with an unspoken emotional positional instruction to the listener of the narrative, the therapist. The expectation would then be that I engage in the discussion of this dream. The unconscious dimension of the narrating self becomes clear: Mrs L. offers Klaus's dream, and I would then "voraciously" digest it, that is, do some "therapeutic work" with it. This dream-telling is a resistance; the dream is offered to me in the form of a sacrifice. I would become the spider and Klaus the victim. This reasoning answers the question of what fear is driving the mother for her to offer me a victim. My answer is that she tends to "claw", not only the dream but also Klaus into her bed.

She took Klaus into her bed, as she now tells us—against Klaus's express wishes! She used him as a kind of "dope" against loneliness in her bed when her husband is absent. She "misused" him, not sexually but in a kind of narcissistic completion. The therapist, in this case, is feared as a strong "over-eye" (Grand, 2013).

After we have been able to talk about this a bit, I point out that the father has hardly said anything so far. Mrs L. says that Klaus had expressed that he knew his mother, but "I don't know Daddy at all." A new unrealised possibility shows up: that one knows the other instead of being "eaten". Mr L. himself does not know who his biological father is. His mother had never told him. He also always had an exclusive relationship with his mother, but he could not make her talk about his father. His long silence in the session up to this point was an enacting of himself as an absent father.

Metaphorical alteration of the couple's past

When I ask how both parents met, Mr L. tells me how he wooed his wife with attractive leisure activities; she says he "bought" her. When I ask if she meant to say that he had also "clawed" her, he starts to cry. He says he never knew what it was like to have a father, and he is shocked by the discovery that he had exposed his son to the same experience of fatherlessness.

This response might be perceived as confusion. In everyday conversation, people's talk is organised partially by sequentiality (one speaker only), by topicality (one topic only), and by complex efforts to override these principles (Schegloff, 2007). However, what we can see here is how a couple goes back into their courting time, creating and exchanging a structuring metaphor (from "buying" to "clawing") and that this metaphoric change is followed by a strong emotional outburst. More than one topic and more than one time level are debated at once, the point of integration of which is the "clawing" metaphor, initially introduced into the dialogue by Klaus's dreamt message.

There is an implicit message in this: the husband agrees that "buying" → "clawing" is a correct description of what he did and how he felt, but the reason for these auxiliary means was that he did not feel like he expected he should have felt. He did not know his father and the expectation to feel and act like a (prospective) father overburdened him. Expressively, we do not hear this confession, but we could be regarded as fools should we not understand it.

Concluding remarks

The interpretation of dreams, we learned from Freud, is the royal road to the unconscious. In the analytic treatment room, dreams are always told under the sign of secrecy. Dream-tellings in the presence of other family members must and should be treated as communication. However, in family therapy, this communication is not only addressed to a single analyst but also told to make something public at the risk of rejecting this communication. Primo Levi told us that the worst thing after surviving Auschwitz was the response of German citizens when he attempted to talk about his experiences. He was again silenced by being told he should be happy to have survived. This response, he wrote, made it gradually impossible for him to continue living (Levi, 1959).

Dreams are risky communications as they can be pushed back in the same or in a similar way. Their message can become silenced again if they fall on a deaf ear. Some people maintain that family members under normal circumstances tell their dreams in the morning at breakfast. However, I do not know of any study that confirms such an assertion.

The general principle holds that every conversation a) is risky, and b) works if a speaker sees a chance to speak to attentively listening ears. To tell "unusual" experiences like a dream is risky when the foray of "daily standard communication in families" is left.

In family therapy sessions, dream-telling appears as a compromise between the first tendency to hold back, which is to keep things silenced, and the second tendency to meet a hearing ear. This offer is the therapist's role and task. His professional task is to listen and to estimate the emotional risk the dream teller runs to tell a dream in the presence of other family members who might respond with intensified efforts to silencing. In my examples, it is the integrative function of the therapist to encourage other family members to hold back familiar responses of silencing the dream teller, and, instead, to open a path for hearing what was silenced and begin to be told during the session.

The understanding of "transmission between generations" can be enriched by studies of non-persecuted families who are nevertheless seriously traumatised—by parental loss, unhappy marriages, attempts to murder, or because they have been genuinely wronged, for example, in inheritance arrangements. I wonder why in family therapy literature questions like those of money, injustice, and heritage are seldom addressed (an exception is Behn et al., 2018). Legal disputes, bitter juridical fights about such issues, are a source of years-long disagreements in the course of which family members inflict serious psychological and sometimes physical injuries on each other.

In families, I tried to show, we encounter equivalences of such traumatic experiences, as it were, "every day". However, they are widely silenced even by the therapeutic community.

It is an important key to understanding the complexity of "normal" family life. I put the word normal in quotation marks because I assume that there is hardly any family without comparable experiences as described here, at least to a minor degree. My examples from my family-therapeutic experience try to show that working with spontaneously reported dreams offers a source of hearing what was silenced.

References

Abraham, K. (1923). The spider as a dream symbol. *International Journal of Psychoanalysis, 4*: 313–317.

Bateson, G. (1978). The birth of a matrix or double bind and epistemology. In: M. M. Berger (Ed.), *Beyond the Double Bind: Communication and Family Systems, Theories and Techniques with Schizophrenics* (pp. 11–36). New York: Brunner/Mazel.

Behn, A. J., Errázuriz, P. A., Cottin, M., & Fischer, C. (2018). Change in symptomatic burden and life satisfaction during short-term psychotherapy: Focusing on the role of family income. *Counselling and Psychotherapy Research, 18*(2): 133–142. https://doi.org/10.1002/capr.12158

Buchholz, M. B. (1982). *Psychoanalytische Methode und Familientherapie.* Frankfurt, Germany: Verlag der psychologischen Fachbuchhandlung.

Buchholz, M. B. (1990a). *Die unbewusste Familie. Psychoanalytische Studien zur Familie in der Moderne (2. Auflage 1995 im Pfeiffer-Verlag).* Berlin: Springer.

Buchholz, M. B. (1990b). Using dreams in family therapy. *Journal of Family Therapy, 12*: 387–396.

Danieli, Y. (2006). It was always there. In: C. R. Figley (Ed.), *Routledge Psychosocial Stress Series: Vol. 31. Mapping Trauma and Its Wake. Autobiographic Essays by Pioneer Trauma Scholars* (pp. 33–46). New York: Routledge.

Deppermann, A., Scheidt, C. E., & Stukenbrock, A. (2020). Positioning shifts: From told self to performative self in psychotherapy. *Frontiers in Psychology, 11.* https://doi.org/10.3389/fpsyg.2020.572436

Gerson, M. J. (1996). *The Embedded Self: A Psychoanalytic Guide to Family Therapy.* Hillsdale, NJ: The Analytic Press.

Graaf, T. K. de (1998). A family therapeutic approach to transgenerational traumatization. *Family Process, 37*: 233–243.

Grand, S. (2013). *The Reproduction of Evil: A Clinical and Cultural Perspective. Relational Perspectives Book Series.* Hoboken, NJ: Taylor & Francis. Retrieved from http://gbv.eblib.com/patron/FullRecord.aspx?p=1222960

Levi, P. (1959). *If This Is a Man*. Stuart Woolf (Trans.). New York: Orion.

Rohde-Dachser, C. (2016). Dem Ungesagten eine Gestalt verleihen. Repräsentationen des Weiblichen in den Kulturproduktionen der Postmoderne. *Zeitschrift für Sexualforschung*, *29*(3): 270–284. https://doi.org/10.1055/s-0042-114413

Schegloff, E. A. (2007). *Sequence Organization in Interaction. A Primer in Conversation Analysis I*. Cambridge: Cambridge University Press.

CHAPTER 12

First-person narratives of madness: the revenge of the silenced

Gail A. Hornstein

Psychiatry has a peculiar history compared with the rest of medicine, partly because it is so closely tied to a particular institution, the asylum, a world where patients have always been as present as physicians. Madness has existed throughout human history, but there was no organised field of psychiatry before the eighteenth century, when what Foucault called "the great confinement" began to spread across parts of Europe. And it was within these mental institutions—regardless of whether they were large public hospitals or small private madhouses—that a new kind of physician, the "alienist", was created, whose job it was to restore lost minds to health. Throughout the next 150 years, psychiatry was defined primarily as the work of caring for these institutionalised patients, the "alienated". This created an intimacy between doctors and patients—who often literally lived together in isolated geographical locations in the same buildings or on the same grounds—that was unique in medicine.

Forced to try to make sense of a strange world that few outside it could even imagine, doctors and patients both took to writing accounts of their asylum experiences. Some speculated about the causes of mental illness or recounted a treatment they had witnessed. Patients often wrote to protest involuntary confinement or to expose deplorable conditions. There are more than 1,000 published patient narratives of madness in English alone (the earliest from 1436); no one knows how many other such accounts remain unpublished, written in other languages, or buried, unacknowledged, in doctors' case records. I have spent many years trying to make these patient narratives better known, often against the resistance of psychiatrists. But at some level, I have always understood their choosing to ignore—if not actively suppress—these accounts, as so many of them cast their profession in a poor light. When I began this work, I didn't realise how many different ways psychiatrists would figure out to keep their patients silenced, some of which I describe in this chapter.

First-person narratives of madness are a kind of protest literature, like slave narratives or witness testimonies. They retell the history of psychiatry as a story of patients struggling to escape the despair of their doctors, to analyse or make public their experiences, and to create alternative forms of healing for themselves.

As editors Jeffrey Geller and Maxine Harris (1994) ask in the introduction to their important collection, *Women of the Asylum: Voices from Behind the Walls, 1840–1945*: "After all, what is a first-person account, but a case study written by the patient rather than the doctor?" The literary critic Mary Elene Wood calls such accounts "life writing" to highlight their creation "across a range of genres—memoir, autobiographical fiction, autobiography, case study", and I agree with this framing. As Wood (2013) notes, it explicitly challenges the standard assumption by doctors that patients, especially those with a psychotic diagnosis, cannot "tell a coherent story", or be reliable (i.e. truthful) narrators. "Their story-telling", Wood continues, "becomes suspect and opaque from the moment of diagnosis; their own words have meaning primarily as symptoms of a mental illness with a grim prognosis." Not only does this pathologise practically every aspect of a patient's experience, but as Wood emphasises, "Diagnosis is a narrative that circumscribes and predicts the future, foreshadowing the course of a particular mental illness in the form of a prognosis, which is usually poor in the case of psychosis."

Preventing patients from speaking

Efforts to silence patients' voices take many forms, both explicit and implicit. To begin with, by allowing patients into the psychological literature only as case illustrations, never as authors, doctors severely restrict the audience for patients' works. Indeed, Wood concludes that one reason there are so many hundreds of first-person accounts in psychiatry—in striking contrast to any other field of medicine—is that these patients must "constantly and repeatedly create life stories over and against psychiatric and popular representations of their experience".

The historian of medicine Roy Porter—one of few in his field to highlight the extent and importance of first-person madness narratives—suggests (2006) that if we stand back from the tired debates among psychiatrists about mind vs brain, we see that a much broader struggle has been going on between doctors and patients regarding madness and its treatment. There have always been patients with distinctive, well-formulated ideas about the mind or nuanced understandings of therapeutic effectiveness. Doctors' viewpoints, of course, have always been privileged over rival accounts by patients, not so much because they are more insightful as because doctors are in charge. As the seventeenth-century playwright Nathaniel Lee wryly remarked as he was being led away to Bethlem Hospital in London: "They called me mad, and I called them mad, and damn them, they outvoted me."

But psychiatrists have not simply ignored patient voices; they have gone to considerable lengths to silence them. Accounts by former patients are filled with reports of being gagged, kept in isolation rooms, threatened with violence for speaking out, drugged to the point where speech was impossible, or having significant chunks of memory erased by ECT. And there is a distressing plethora of forms of silencing less literal than these, but no less destructive.

In a famous scene in Mary Jane Ward's autobiographical novel *The Snake Pit*, published in 1946, the main character opens her mouth to call for a lawyer to protest being forcibly administered shock treatment. A nurse thrusts a gag into her open mouth, saying, "Thank you, dear," apparently assuming the patient was trying to be cooperative. Elizabeth Packard, the author of the 1874 classic *Modern Persecution*, or *Insane Asylums Unveiled*, had to pencil her notes into the cotton undergarments the nurses allowed her to embroider, which her children then smuggled off the ward. Daniel Paul Schreber's physician filed a court order to block the appearance of his 1903 *Memoirs of My Nervous Illness*, arguing that Schreber's desire to publish was just another of his symptoms. Administrators of English asylums routinely destroyed letters written by patients; the Lunacy Act of 1890 had categorised them as "insane literature".

Charlotte Perkins Gilman, the great nineteenth-century economist and feminist theorist, recounts in her barely fictionalised short story *The Yellow Wallpaper* (1892) how she was imprisoned in a nursery for the so-called "rest cure" and forbidden even to write in her journal. She bitterly recalls her doctor's warning "never [to] touch pen, brush, or pencil as long as you live", and says in her autobiography (1935) that obeying his injunction brought her "perilously near" to losing her mind entirely. After months of crawling under beds and into closets "to hide from the grinding power of that profound distress", Gilman finally began to write again and cured herself.

Lori Schiller, a patient in various New York mental institutions in the 1970s, had to enlist family members and friends to write some of the chapters in her memoir, *The Quiet Room* (Schiller & Bennett, 1994), because of the heavy doses of medication and ECT she was prescribed. "They had electrocuted the memories right out of me ... taken away big chunks of my life," she later commented bitterly.

Porter emphasises that patients were silenced regardless of who they were. John Perceval, son of a prime minister, was a patient in the 1830s at several asylums for England's wealthy. In his famous first-person account *Narrative of the Treatment Received by a Gentleman*, Perceval declares that despite the elegant surroundings, he was treated "as if I were a piece of furniture, an image of wood, incapable of desire or will as well as judgement". He found it insulting that even though he had an educated and aristocratic background, he "was not once addressed by argument, expostulation, or persuasion", and that his doctors lied to him, opened his letters, and denied him writing materials. Kate Millet, the renowned feminist writer and activist, recounts in her memoir, *The Loony-Bin Trip* (1990), how she was incarcerated in the 1980s in several institutions in the US and Ireland against her strenuous objections after refusing to take prescribed medications that had caused unbearable side effects.

Agnes Richter, the title character of my book *Agnes's Jacket: A Psychologist's Search for the Meanings of Madness* (2018), was forcibly institutionalised in Dresden, Germany, in the 1890s. She managed to tell her story only through a coded autobiographical text embroidered into a garment she fashioned out of a hospital uniform. Her elaborate and beautiful stitching, and the urgency of her words, repeatedly stabbed into the cloth, are evidence of a double silencing—the refusal of her doctors to listen, and Agnes's self-censorship, from fear or suspicion, thereby leaving the message of the jacket opaque and largely incomprehensible.

Refusing to take first-person accounts seriously

As filmmaker and former patient Allie Light writes, the dismissal of patient experience can sometimes go to absurd lengths. Light (1999) describes the time in the early 1960s when she and her psychiatrist were walking down a hall at the hospital where she was then a patient. "We were just about to enter the ward, when a young man, another patient, came running toward us. He was agitated, frantic, and frenzied, and he carried the receiver of the wall telephone in his hand. He had jerked it off the wall. When he saw the doctor, he began to shout, 'The president is dead. He's been killed. The president has been shot.' The doctor turned to me and said, 'Don't pay any attention to him, he's just hallucinating.' That was the assassination of John F. Kennedy."

The question of who gets to tell the story of how the mind works has long been particularly important and charged in psychiatry, far more than in other fields of medicine. *How* an experience is described and who gets to describe it largely determine what response will follow. Since treatments in psychiatry are developed primarily through trial and error, and less often in laboratories than through case management, the power of rhetoric often becomes more important than data.

This is evident in the continuing appeal of biological models of understanding and treating psychological distress, which, despite their limited evidence base, tell a compelling and easy-to-understand story. Any abnormality of experience—regardless of whether it involves thoughts, perceptions, emotions, behavior, etc.—is framed framed as a disorder of genetics or brain chemistry. Nothing else in a person's life has to be considered; it's solely a question of biology. The rhetorical power of this story—for both psychiatrists and patients—makes it seem less like a hypothesis than a fact, effectively silencing alternatives.

But the hegemony of doctors' accounts is not limited to biological explanations. As the patient activist and writer Judi Chamberlin notes, even radical psychiatrists discredit and ignore the views of their patients, albeit in more subtle ways. For example, the British psychiatrist R. D. Laing, who pioneered a phenomenological approach to madness that highlighted the significance of personal experience, nevertheless discounted patients' sense-making. As Chamberlin (1978) puts it, Laing "grants that what 'schizophrenics' say has meaning, but only through his translations". In other words, patients' understandings of their own experience are not what counts; it's the *psychiatrist's framing of their experience* that matters and shapes what happens.

Indeed, it's often the *only* thing that matters. Because psychiatrists are among the few physicians routinely allowed to force treatment on their patients, they have a more urgent need to control the narrative of what is happening and prevent alternative ways of making sense of the situation. They must present treatment decisions—especially if they go against the will of the patient—as being based on sound medical knowledge. Yet psychiatrists are at a huge disadvantage as compared to their colleagues in other fields of medicine in establishing their claims as authoritative. Since there are no biological tests, scans, assays, or measurements that they can use to support the diagnosis of a mental illness, psychiatrists have to rely on their powers of persuasion. But their treatment methods remain controversial and often cause debilitating side effects or fail to work, so they end up with a stark choice—either push patients (and their families) to accept a biological explanation of their problem and the treatments that are derived from it or, if necessary, force it upon them.

Silencing solidarity

Patients in psychiatric hospitals face a different form of silencing, the silencing of solidarity. In many institutions, patients who have been released are not permitted to contact those still on the ward, thereby preventing friendships from continuing or developing. During group meetings in clinical contexts, "crosstalk", that is, normal human dialogue, is often explicitly prohibited. Patients are allowed to speak in the group only when a staff facilitator calls on them; direct interchange between patients is discouraged. Chamberlin tells the story of a group of ex-patients in Vancouver, British Columbia, in the early 1970s, who had to circulate a list of each other's phone numbers secretly so they could support one another without the staff finding out and stopping it.

Psychiatric mystification

Chamberlin describes another form of silencing, which she calls "psychiatric mystification". By deliberately using vague and euphemistic terms, the realities of what transpires in a mental institution are disguised or hidden. Isolation cells become "seclusion rooms" or the yet more innocuous-sounding "quiet rooms"; drugs are "medications"; straitjackets are "camisoles"; coercion, restraint, involuntary ECT, etc. are "treatments"; and wearing one's own clothes, being able to go outside, etc. are "privileges". At the broadest level, problems in living become "mental illnesses".

Distorting patient experience in the service of theory

Some doctors openly distort their patients' experiences to fit their frameworks—yet another form of silencing. For example, the demure, obedient "Eve White" was hailed as the "real" personality of the patient in the classic book and film *The Three Faces of Eve*, with the sexy, outspoken "Eve Black" banished during therapy. (Years later, the patient retaliated by publishing her own book, *I'm Eve* [Sizemore & Pittillo, 1977], exposing the extent of her doctors' manipulation.) Freud so appropriated Schreber's story that it wasn't until 1955 when *Memoirs of My Nervous Illness* was translated into English and republished, that readers could compare the patient's 1903 original with Freud's 1911 version. Then they could see for themselves how Freud's narrow use of the case to prove his theory that paranoia is caused by repressed homosexuality required a massive rewriting of Schreber's experience.

Patients' complaints about being unheard are often dismissed as evidence of their illness. As Mary Jane Ward acidly remarked of her asylum psychiatrist: "He [was] always talking about hearing voices, and never hearing mine."

Clarissa Caldwell Lathrop, who spent two years at the New York State Lunatic Asylum at Utica between 1880 and 1882, recalled (Lathrop, 1890): "I learned that it was not best to allow anyone to see me weep, lest it might be said in addition to their former absurd statements [about me] that I was a victim of Melancholia." In other words, in an asylum, even crying could be silenced to ensure a patient's compliance and avoid additional diagnoses.

Silencing by stigma

Silencing can take both outer and inner forms. Howard Dully, for example, recalls how several years after his lobotomy, "I began to disappear from family photos." This *outer* silencing followed decades of *inner* silencing. Dully's lobotomy took place in 1960 when he was twelve years old. For the next forty years, he says he was "haunted" by the question: "Was there something I had done and forgotten—something so horrible that I deserved a lobotomy?" This question was so shaming that Dully says, "although I thought about my lobotomy all the time, I never talked about it. It was my terrible secret. What was so *wrong* with me?" (Dully & Fleming, 2007).

The reason we know any of this now is that in 2007, Dully published, with a journalist co-author, a book-length memoir, *My Lobotomy*, recounting his experiences. He decided to do so after giving an emotional interview to two radio producers who brought his story to a national US audience; listeners were so powerfully affected by the broadcast that their massive influx of emails crashed the network's server.

Family members of psychiatric patients are also silenced by stigma and stereotypes about mental illness. They worry about what relatives, co-workers, and neighbours might think (and they are right to do so, given the persistence of popular fears about violent or uncontrollable mental patients). Howard Dully's erasure from family photos might seem extreme, but many families resort to silence about their relatives who are patients. Asylums often underscored this silencing by burying those who died in the institution in unmarked graves (so as not to "shame" families).

Challenging credibility

Like slave narratives, accounts by psychiatric patients often pit the experience of one person against a broader social structure perceived as oppressive and unjust. Realising that readers are likely to be sceptical, patients struggle to establish themselves as reliable narrators. Some have a psychiatrist or other authority write a foreword to increase the credibility of their books. Others use statistics or report on the experiences of many different patients to buttress their arguments for reform. Those who recognise that their experiences challenge standard psychiatric practice may make explicit comparisons to doctors' views. John Custance, for example, in his 1952 book *Wisdom, Madness and Folly*, analysed his symptoms in relation to Freud's and Jung's theories of the unconscious, Kant's epistemology, Nietzsche's principle of opposites, and Goethe's Faust. (An Oxford professor of philosophy contributed a highly laudatory preface to Custance's work.) The dancer Vaslav Nijinsky, frustrated by his doctor's lack of imagination and narrowness of thought, confided to his diary (1936): "He wants to examine my brain. I want to examine his mind."

Even patients who find their treatment helpful may still feel an acute desire to tell their story on their own terms. Marie Cardinal, for example, despite being a celebrated writer, nevertheless titled her "autobiographical novel" *The Words to Say It* (1983) because she felt compelled to situate the psychoanalysis that dramatically cured her of madness within a broader life and historical narrative that her Parisian analyst simply could not grasp (especially relating to her youth as a young French girl in war-torn Algeria).

Silencing culture

What global health scholars Francisco Ortega and Leandro David Wenceslau call the "silencing of culture" is widespread in psychiatry. Cultural factors and explanations of the causes and outcomes of mental distress are ignored, and this "misrecognition of the cultural dimension within mental health practices and interventions ... [is] underpinned by frequent contempt for popular beliefs and culture. The most obvious example of this silencing is the issue of religious beliefs and practices and their role within mental health services and interventions." As Ortega and Wenceslau's analysis (2020) shows: "Mental health professionals tend to adopt reductionist views of the relationship between religious beliefs and behaviours and mental distress and often disregard users' religious experience as significant to the cause, course, and outcome of their distress."

This is clearly seen among patients who hear voices. Throughout history, people have reported unusual perceptions or intense emotions during spiritual experiences. Most of the major religions of the world revere key figures who heard celestial voices speaking to them. Yet people who end up in the psychiatric system and frame their voice-hearing experiences within a context of spirituality are typically pathologised as delusional. And whether or not their voices are religious, all voice hearers are silenced by the standard psychiatric practice of not asking anything about what the voices are saying, instead encouraging patients to try to block out or ignore them.

Delegitimising specific forms of suffering

Meri Nana-Ama Danquah shows how the specific nature of what is silenced in a patient's experience can vary widely across subcultures. Some patients have their strength and resilience rendered invisible by assumptions of inherent vulnerability. But for black women, it can be just the opposite. As Danquah (1998) writes: "The illusion of strength has been and continues to be of major significance to me as a black woman. The one myth I have had to endure my entire life is that of my supposed birthright to strength. Black women are *supposed* to be strong— caretakers, nurturers, healers of other people ... Emotional hardship is *supposed* to be built into the structure of our lives." So, paradoxically, Danquah's deep depression and feelings of helplessness—which might readily have been recognised as problems in a white woman—remained unseen and unheard by a racist mental health system.

She highlights a further kind of silencing, evident in metaphoric depictions of depression, which routinely equate depression with "blackness" as a symbol of badness—"a black hole; an enveloping darkness; a dismal existence through which no light shines; the black dog; darkness, and more darkness. But what does darkness mean to me," Danquah asks, "a woman who has spent her life surrounded by it?

The darkness of my skin; the darkness of my friends and family. I have never been afraid of the dark. It poses no harm to me. What is the colour of *my* depression?" At the same time, she says, "I didn't want my depression to be the only thing that defined or distinguished me."

Diagnosis as identity

Indeed, this is another form of silencing faced by psychiatric patients—turning a diagnosis into the key factor defining a person's identity. This doesn't typically happen with diagnoses of physical illnesses—we say "I *have* cancer or heart disease or diabetes" not "I *am* cancer or heart disease, etc." But people with psychiatric diagnoses are often reduced to their supposed illness—"he's schizophrenic", or she's "bipolar" or "borderline", etc. Even those who manage to get better often have the rest of their lives framed as "recovery" or "remission", not simply as human existence, with all the complexity and variability inherent in it for anyone.

Undermining historians' attempts to highlight patient voices

I was trained as a psychologist, so when I decided I wanted to write about the history of psychology, psychiatry, and psychoanalysis, I gladly accepted an invitation to spend a year as a visiting fellow in a prominent history of science department. Practitioners who write histories of their disciplines are often (rightly) critiqued for indulging in polemic rather than systematic analyses of primary source materials. I wanted historians of science and medicine to take my work seriously, so I immersed myself in their field—participating in graduate seminars and research groups; attending and speaking at the meetings of their professional associations; reviewing manuscripts for their publications; and seeking the guidance of senior colleagues as I developed my own research interests. They encouraged me at every turn, supported my applications for grants to fund this work, and applauded the publication of my first book, the biography of a pioneering psychiatrist (*To Redeem One Person Is to Redeem the World: The Life of Frieda Fromm-Reichmann*, 2000).

So, I was surprised and dismayed when, embarking on the research for my second project, I found these same colleagues responding to the work with disbelief and discouragement. What had changed? Mainly, my source of data—instead of relying on the accounts of physicians (whose diagnostic categories, theories, treatments, and case records constitute the primary sources for most work in the history of medicine), I was using the accounts of patients (typically dismissed as "biased" and considered especially unreliable in psychiatry, where patients are assumed to be "out of touch with reality"). In other words, instead of writing medical history (i.e. analysing the actions and changing beliefs of doctors), I was resorting to politics (i.e. analysing the actions and changing beliefs of patients, which doctors considered "symptoms" rather than substantive contributions). To take seriously the critiques, theoretical frameworks, and therapeutic alternatives proposed by psychiatric patients was, I was told, tantamount to "going native", as anthropologists call the "error" of taking on the viewpoints of those they study. My work was no longer seen as "objective"—so, I realised, not only were patients themselves being silenced in all the ways described above but historians who sought to rely on their accounts as primary source materials were themselves silenced by being seen as violating the values of distanced, dispassionate research that would allow their conclusions to be taken as valid.

This ignoring or minimising the contributions of patients is particularly unfortunate in psychiatry, given how little is understood about emotional distress and how urgent the need for help continues to be. Besides being anti-democratic, it robs the field of an important source of alternative theories and methods. Innovations like the Hearing Voices approach, which emerged directly from voice-hearers themselves and has now spread to thirty countries on five continents, is a vivid contemporary example of the innovative and effective frameworks that people with first-hand experience of psychosis can contribute to psychiatry.

At the broadest level, patient narratives provide an extraordinary insight into the phenomenology of psychosis and the ways that patients experience or interpret treatments of various kinds. They focus our attention on the contexts (political, historical, cultural, economic, familial) within which emotional distress arises, rather than on the "defects" or "disease entities" internal to the patient which doctors typically describe. Patient narratives also force us to revise some of our core assumptions about psychiatry's history and goals and demonstrate that some of the best-known "cures" claimed by psychiatrists turn out to be exaggerations or myths. Within psychoanalytic history, for example, recently discovered data on such key patients as Breuer's Anna O.,

Jung's Sabina Spielrein, and Ferenczi's Elizabeth Severn (hidden behind the code "RN" in his "Clinical Diary") show that it was they—not their doctors—who introduced such technical innovations as "catharsis", "mutual analysis", and "active imagination".

The multiple forms of silencing that I have described here—preventing patients from speaking; refusing to publish or take seriously what they say; delegitimising specific forms of suffering; undermining historians' attempts to highlight patient voices, etc.—have all been extraordinarily effective in keeping first-person accounts of madness largely invisible and unheard. But the constantly increasing number of such accounts, and the new means by which they can now be circulated and read—via self-publishing, or on websites, or in oral histories or blogs—suggests that such silencing can never fully succeed and is becoming less and less successful. Indeed, against all odds, and even though the very existence of these works seems impossible—doesn't madness preclude a coherent account of itself?—narratives by psychiatric patients form a unique kind of literature that for hundreds of years has sought to break through all efforts at silencing.

Endnote

My Bibliography of First-Person Madness Narratives, now in its fifth edition, lists more than 1,000 published accounts in English and is available for free download from my website: www.gailhornstein.com/works.htm. A published version of the fourth edition can also be found in: G. Eghigian (Ed.), *From Madness to Mental Health: Psychiatric Disorder and Its Treatment in Western Civilization*. New Brunswick, NJ: Rutgers University Press, 2010.

References

Cardinal, M. (1983). *The Words to Say It*. Cambridge, MA: VanVactor & Goodheart.

Chamberlin, J. (1978). *On Our Own: Patient-Controlled Alternatives to the Mental Health System*. New York: McGraw-Hill.

Custance, J. (1952). *Wisdom, Madness and Folly: The Philosophy of a Lunatic*. New York: Pellegrini & Cudahy.

Danquah, M. N.-A. (1998). *Willow Weep for Me: A Black Woman's Journey Through Depression*. New York: One World/Ballantine.

Dully, H., & Fleming, C. (2007). *My Lobotomy: A Memoir*. New York: Crown.

Geller, J. L., & Harris, M. (Eds.) (1994). *Women of the Asylum: Voices from Behind the Walls, 1840–1945*. New York: Anchor/Doubleday.

Gilman, C. P. (1892). *The Yellow Wallpaper*. New York: The Feminist Press, 1973.

Gilman, C. P. (1935). *The Living of Charlotte Perkins Gilman: An Autobiography*. New York: Appleton-Century.

Hornstein, G. A. (2000). *To Redeem One Person Is to Redeem the World: The Life of Frieda Fromm-Reichmann*. New York: Free Press/Simon & Schuster.

Hornstein, G. A. (2009). *Agnes's Jacket: A Psychologist's Search for the Meanings of Madness*. New York: Rodale (revised edition, Routledge, 2018).

Lathrop, C. C. (1890). A secret institution. Excerpted in J. L. Geller & M. Harris (Eds.), *Women of the Asylum: Voices from Behind the Walls, 1840–1945*. New York: Anchor Books/Doubleday, 1994.

Light, A. (1999). Thorazine shuffle. In: R. Shannonhouse (Ed.), *Out of Her Mind: Women Writing on Madness*. New York: Modern Library, 2000.

Millet, K. (1990). *The Loony-Bin Trip*. New York: Simon & Schuster.

Nijinsky, V. (1936). *The Diary of Vaslav Nijinsky*. New York: Farrar, Straus & Giroux, 1999.

Ortega, F., & Wenceslau, L. D. (2020). Challenges for implementing a global mental health agenda in Brazil: The "silencing" of culture. *Transcultural Psychiatry, 57*: 57–70.

Packard, E. (1874). *Modern Persecution or Insane Asylums Unveiled*. Hartford, CT: Self-published.

Perceval, J. (1838). *A Narrative of the Treatment Received by a Gentleman, During a State of Mental Derangement*. London: Effingham Wilson.

Porter, R. (2006). *Madmen: A Social History of Madhouses, Mad-Doctors & Lunatics*. Stroud, UK: Tempus.

Schiller, L., & Bennett, A. (1994). *The Quiet Room: A Journey Out of the Torment of Madness*. New York: Warner.

Schreber, D. P. (1903). *Memoirs of My Nervous Illness*. New York: New York Review of Books, 1955.

Sizemore, C. C., & Pittillo, E. S. (1977). *I'm Eve*. New York: Doubleday.

Ward, M. J. (1946). *The Snake Pit*. New York: Random House.

Wood, M. E. (2013). *Life Writing and Schizophrenia: Encounters at the Edge of Meaning*. Amsterdam, the Netherlands: Rodopi.

Index